FOOD IRRADIATION
A technique for preserving and improving the safety of food

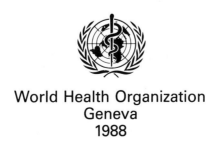

World Health Organization
Geneva
1988

ISBN 92 4 154240 3

© WORLD HEALTH ORGANIZATION 1988

Publications of the World Health Organization enjoy copyright protection in accordance with the provisions of Protocol 2 of the Universal Copyright Convention. For rights of reproduction or translation of WHO publications, in part or *in toto,* application should be made to the Office of Publications, World Health Organization, Geneva, Switzerland. The World Health Organization welcomes such applications.

The designations employed and the presentation of the material in this publication do not imply the expression of any opinion whatsoever on the part of the Secretariat of the World Health Organization concerning the legal status of any country, territory, city or area or of its authorities, or concerning the delimitation of its frontiers or boundaries.

The mention of specific companies or of certain manufacturers' products does not imply that they are endorsed or recommended by the World Health Organization in preference to others of a similar nature that are not mentioned. Errors and omissions excepted, the names of proprietary products are distinguished by initial capital letters.

Printed in Switzerland

88/7649—Phototypesetting—6000

CONTENTS

	Page
Preface	5
Acknowledgements	6
Introduction	8
1. Established methods of food processing	11
2. The process of food irradiation	18
3. Effects of food irradiation	24
4. Practical applications of food irradiation	33
5. Legislation and control of food irradiation	44
6. Consumer acceptance	48
Bibliography	56
Annex 1. List of countries that have cleared irradiated food for human consumption	62
Annex 2. Codex General Standard for Irradiated Foods	72
Annex 3. Recommended International Code of Practice for the Operation of Irradiation Facilities Used for the Treatment of Food	75

PREFACE

One of the common objectives of the Food and Agriculture Organization of the United Nations and the World Health Organization is to assist the efforts of individual governments throughout the world to provide safe and nutritious food supplies. This book has been prepared to help achieve that objective. Its aim is to provide a factual comprehensive review of the role of food irradiation in controlling two of the most serious problems connected with food supplies: the huge avoidable losses of food through deterioration and the illness and death that result from the use of contaminated food.

The book is not a technical treatise. Instead, it is intended to provide basic information for general readers, students, policy-makers, consumers, and the media, concerning the nature of food irradiation and its effects on food, its benefits and disadvantages, and, perhaps most important of all, its safety. Those seeking more extensive scientific information, such as reports on the safety of irradiated food or technical descriptions of food irradiation processes, should consult the extensive bibliography at the end of the book.

Decades of study and practical application have fostered increasing confidence in the ability of food irradiation to protect and preserve food and thereby to safeguard health. Misconceptions abound, however, about whether irradiated food is safe to eat and how irradiation can complement or replace other methods of preserving foods. This book is an attempt to correct those misconceptions and to help people in all parts of the world make sound decisions about the place of food irradiation in their efforts to secure an adequate, wholesome, and dependable food supply.

In publishing this book, the two Organizations do not wish to give the idea that food irradiation is a panacea for all the numerous food supply problems in the world, but rather to provide reassurance that the process may, under certain circumstances, be safely used to improve food safety, to reduce food losses, and to facilitate food trade. The Organizations are indeed concerned that the unwarranted criticism of the process may hamper its use in the countries that may benefit most.

ACKNOWLEDGEMENTS

In the production of this book, FAO and WHO have been guided by an editorial board, composed of the following:

Professor E.H. Kampelmacher, National Institute of Public Health and Environmental Hygiene, Bilthoven, The Netherlands (*Chairman*);

Professor M.J. Rand, Department of Pharmacology, The University of Melbourne, Parkville, Victoria, Australia;

Mrs M. Young, Food Policy Committee, Consumers Association of Canada, Ontario, Canada;

Dr B. Chinsman, United Nations Development Programme, United Nations Fund for Science and Technology for Development, New York, USA (formerly, Director, African Regional Centre for Technology, Dakar, Senegal).

The text of the book is based on contributions from the following:

Dr B. Chinsman (address as above);

Professor J.F. Diehl, Federal Research Institute for Nutrition, Karlsruhe, Federal Republic of Germany;

Dr Ronald E. Engel, Food Safety and Inspection Service, US Department of Agriculture, Washington, DC, USA;

Dr J. Farkas, Central Food Research Institute, Budapest, Hungary;

Dr Y. Henon, Aix-en-Provence, France;

Professor C.H. Mannheim, Department of Food Engineering and Biotechnology, Israel Institute of Technology, Haifa, Israel;

W.M. Urbain, Professor Emeritus, Department of Food Science and Human Nutrition, Michigan State University, USA;

Mrs M. Young (address as above).

The individual contributions from the various authors were reviewed by the following institutions:

ASEAN Food Handling Bureau, Kuala Lumpur, Malaysia;

Food and Drug Administration, Center for Food Safety and Applied Nutrition, Washington, DC, USA;

Indian National Institute for Nutrition, Hyderabad, India;

Post Harvest Horticultural Laboratory, Department of Agriculture, Gosford, New South Wales, Australia.

The editing and some rewriting of the contributions were undertaken by the Communication Staff of the US Food and Drug Administration, Rockville, MD, USA. The book was checked for technical accuracy by the Food Preservation Section, Joint FAO/IAEA Division, at the International Atomic Energy Agency, Vienna, and also by the WHO units concerned with Radiation Medicine and Prevention of Environmental Pollution, Geneva, Switzerland.

Scientific coordination was assured by Dr F.K. Käferstein, Manager, Food Safety, WHO, Geneva, Switzerland.

INTRODUCTION

In every part of the world people wage a constant battle against the spoilage of food caused by infestation, contamination, and deterioration. There are no exact data on how much of the world's food supply is spoiled, but losses are enormous, especially in developing countries where, often, a warm climate favours the growth of spoilage organisms and hastens the deterioration of stored food. In such countries, the estimated storage loss of cereal grains and legumes is at least 10%. With non-grain staples, vegetables, and fruits, the losses due to microbial contamination and spoilage are believed to be as high as 50%. In commodities such as dried fish, insect infestation is reported to result in the loss of 25% of the product, plus an additional 10% loss due to spoilage. With a rapidly expanding world population, any preventable loss of food is intolerable.

However, the loss of edible food is only part of a larger problem. In 1983 a Joint FAO/WHO Expert Committee on Food Safety[1] concluded that foodborne disease, while not well documented, was one of the most widespread threats to human health and an important cause of reduced economic productivity. A relatively high percentage of raw foods of animal origin are contaminated by pathogenic bacteria, and this results in high levels of foodborne illness in all countries for which statistics are available. Among the factors that appear to account for the increases in foodborne disease are explosive growth in the mass rearing of food animals, polluted environments, mass production of foods of plant origin, increasing international trade in food and animal feed, and the large-scale movement of people as guest workers, immigrants, and tourists.

Meat and meat products also play a major role in infections such as trichinosis and toxoplasmosis, caused by a parasitic nematode (or worm) and a protozoon-like microorganism respectively. It is conservatively estimated that the cost of medical care and lost productivity resulting from major diseases spread by contaminated meat and poultry amounts to at least US$ 1000 million a year in the United States of America alone.

Efforts to reduce the devastating consequences of food wastage and foodborne disease started before the first written records. Probably the first method ever used, and one still widely employed throughout the world today, was sun-drying — simple, cheap, and often highly effective. In the course of tens of thousands of years,

---

[1] WHO Technical Report Series, No. 705, 1984.

people have discovered many other methods of preserving food — salting, cooking, smoking, canning, freezing, and chemical preservation. The most recent addition to this list is irradiation, i.e., the exposure of foods to carefully measured amounts of ionizing radiation. Research and practical application over several decades have shown that irradiation can retard food spoilage and reduce infestation by insects and/or contamination by other organisms, including those that cause foodborne diseases.

Public acceptance of the concept of food irradiation has been less than enthusiastic in some countries. Fears of thermonuclear war and accidents such as those at Three Mile Island in the USA and Chernobyl in the USSR have made many people apprehensive about the use of nuclear energy for any purpose, even one as obviously desirable as improving the quantity and quality of food. Such apprehension is often based on lack of information and confusion between the process of irradiation and contamination with radioactivity. Even in some parts of the world where food irradiation has been employed for many years, members of the public and those who influence public opinion are often not well informed about the process. As noted in the preface, this book has been prepared to help narrow that information gap.

Chapter 1 provides information about the established and widely used methods of preserving and safeguarding our food supply, and should help the reader understand the role that irradiation can play. The first chapter serves as background for the description in Chapter 2 of the origins and development of food irradiation. Chapter 3 presents information on the effects of irradiation on food and on the safety and quality of irradiated food, which are the areas of greatest concern, confusion, and misunderstanding.

Chapter 4 is an introduction to the methods of food irradiation being used today in various countries and the results achieved. It indicates which foodstuffs are suitable for radiation treatment, what actually happens to food and food contaminants when they are subjected to ionizing radiation, and what levels of radiation are used to preserve various kinds of food. This chapter also reviews special problems, such as those faced by tropical and developing countries, that must be addressed in any consideration of the use of food irradiation.

Chapter 5 provides information on the types of legislation required to control the setting-up and operation of food irradiation facilities. The regulations should indicate which foods may be treated, the doses that may be employed to achieve specific effects, and what information must be included in the labelling. The important topics of quality control, inspection, and safety of the public and the operators are also dealt with briefly.

Finally, Chapter 6 takes up the critical issue of consumer acceptance. Through a series of questions that consumers and consumer organizations have raised about food irradiation, and concise factual answers to those questions, this chapter focuses on the need for public understanding as the only reliable path towards greater acceptance and fuller use of food irradiation for the benefit of mankind.

The scientific and technical literature on each of these topics is far too extensive to be treated thoroughly in this publication. Readers who want more detailed information are strongly encouraged to refer to the bibliography at the end of the book, which covers most of the subjects dealt with and provides a useful guide to further reading. Three annexes are appended to the text: Annex 1 gives a list of countries in which irradiation is permitted as a method of food processing; the Codex General Standard for Irradiated Foods is reproduced in Annex 2; and the Recommended International Code of Practice for the Operation of Irradiation Facilities Used for the Treatment of Food is reproduced in Annex 3.

Chapter 1
ESTABLISHED METHODS OF FOOD PROCESSING

The techniques used for preserving food vary from comparatively simple methods, such as sun-drying, to highly sophisticated processes requiring complex equipment and specially trained personnel. To appreciate how food irradiation fits into this spectrum, it is helpful to have a basic understanding of the traditional methods of food preservation — those surviving from antiquity, as well as those that are the fruits of modern science.

The ability to preserve food helped make civilization possible. Once primitive people had discovered how to keep food for relatively long periods, they could give up the pattern of ceaseless wandering in search of an adequate food supply. They could plant, raise, and harvest enough food to last until the next harvest and, when necessary, to sustain them through times of low food production. The discovery that food could be processed and preserved enabled human beings to establish settled communities and to live in ways not so very different from the way most people live today.

The use of fire for food preservation can be traced to the pre-Neolithic period. Other methods — salting, smoking, drying, fermentation, and freezing — are known to have been used by Neolithic people 10 000 or more years ago. Sun-dried fruits were highly prized in the countries around the Mediterranean Sea in ancient times, and potato-drying was practised in South America many centuries before the rise of the Inca empire. The Indians of pre-Colombian North America used air-drying, with or without smoking, to preserve deer and buffalo meat. Fish were dried, salted, and smoked on the shores of the North Atlantic, and both meat and fish were preserved by freezing in cold climates.

These early peoples did not understand, however, why drying, smoking, freezing, and other methods prevented food from going bad. The role of microbes in food spoilage was not discovered until the time of Pasteur. But even without a scientific basis, human ingenuity produced sophisticated food-processing techniques. The first successful process for preserving food by heating it in a suitable container that was then tightly sealed was discovered at the time of the Napoleonic Wars in the early 19th century. Indeed, war has played a significant role in the evolution of food processing. The American Civil War prompted a major expansion of that country's canning industry, and the Second World War stimulated progress in the dehydration of food. In our own times, the special food storage and handling requirements of manned space exploration have resulted in important developments in the freeze-drying and packaging of food.

The traditional methods of preserving food can be divided into five major groups: fermentation, chemical treatment, drying, heat treatment, and freezing.

Fermentation

Fermentation preserves foods by the selective removal of the fermentable substrate and the consequent development of an unfavourable environment for spoilage organisms. Microorganisms are used to ferment sugars to alcohol or acids. A number of factors determine what kind of product is obtained by fermentation: the kind of organism used, the material being processed, the temperature, and the amount of available oxygen determine whether the end-product of fermentation will be beer, wine, leavened bread, or cheese.

Yeasts are the most efficient microbial converters of sugar to alcohol and are essential for the making of beer and wine. Fermentation that leads to the formation of lactic acid is important in the pickling of vegetables and in the processing of a wide variety of dairy products. Pickling of meat in the presence of salt, nitrates, and smoke is an ancient process that is still being refined and widely used. Modern industrial applications of fermentation demand careful control of the process to ensure high yields, and to maintain a uniform high product quality.

Chemical treatment

Preservation of food by the addition of chemicals is a relatively simple and inexpensive technique. It is especially useful in areas where refrigeration is not readily available. On the other hand, concern about the health risks associated with some of the chemicals traditionally used to preserve food has led some countries to curtail their use or to ban some of them from use in foods.

The substances employed in food preservation are of two general kinds: common food ingredients, such as sugar and salt, and specific substances that prevent or retard food deterioration. In the latter category are the so-called food additives and certain other chemicals of value in lengthening the shelf-life of fresh foods or preventing infestation of grains and other foods during bulk storage.

Sugar in concentrations of 65% or more preserves food by lowering the water activity and hence inhibiting the growth of microorganisms. Products such as fruit preserves, jams, and syrups are commonly processed with sugar. In the modern industrial setting, sugar preservation is often supplemented by the use of heat, cooling, and air-free packaging to help control surface mould formation and to prevent discoloration and loss of flavour. In modern food processing, a non-nutritive sweetener, such as sorbitol, may be used as a substitute for sugar.

The use of salt to cure meat, fish, and vegetables is an ancient practice that is widely, if somewhat differently, applied today. Salt keeps spoilage organisms under control and acts as a drying agent, again by reducing the water activity. It is often combined with use of nitrites and external drying, especially in the preservation of meat and fish. In those products, the destructive action of bacteria and enzymes is retarded. In recent years, changes in taste, combined with growing concern about health hazards associated with a high intake of salt, have led to a significant lessening in the use of salt as a food preservative. Improved sanitation combined with refrigeration can make it less necessary to employ high concentrations of salt to preserve meats, fish, and vegetables.

The preservative action of the smoking of food can be attributed to the combined effect of smoke and heat, or to smoke alone. In any case, while this method of food preservation has been known for centuries, it is used much less today because some of the constituents of smoke are now known to be carcinogenic. Liquid substitutes are increasingly being employed to impart a smoked flavour to foods.

Among the food additives approved for use as chemical preservatives in many countries are propionic acid, benzoic acid, sorbic acid, and their salts and derivatives. Sulfur dioxide and sulfites have a long history as important preservative agents, but recently their use has been severely limited in several countries because of health concerns. All these substances are most effective in foods that are dry or fairly acidic; they are of limited or no value in watery low-acid foods, such as mushrooms and certain green vegetables. In addition to its wide use in beverages, carbon dioxide at higher than normal atmospheric pressure can help retard the maturation of some fresh fruits and maintain the quality of fresh meats, fish, poultry, baked goods, and salads. Carbon dioxide extends shelf-life and is relatively inexpensive, although refrigeration is required in addition for foods of animal origin.

Several other chemicals, notably methyl bromide, ethylene dibromide, and ethylene oxide, have been widely used as antimicrobial agents and as fumigants to destroy insects in various foods, such as spices, copra, and walnuts. Evidence that ethylene dibromide and ethylene oxide are harmful to man has led to their being banned by some national regulatory authorities in the last few years. The use of other fumigants is also under review because of the potential dangers to human beings and the environment.

Drying

In addition to protecting perishable foods against deterioration, drying offers other important advantages. The removal of water reduces both the weight and the bulk of food products and thus lowers transportation and storage costs. Dehydration can also make foods suitable for subsequent processing that may, in turn, facilitate handling, packaging, shipping, and consumption. Both physical and chemical changes take place during food drying, but not all of them are desirable. In addition to changes in bulk density, foods may undergo unwelcome colour changes, such as browning; they may also lose nutritional value, flavour, and even the capacity to re-absorb water.

Successful food dehydration depends on the correct selection of the method and equipment to be used. That depends on the type of food to be dried, what properties the final product must have, and the size and capacity of the processing unit. The most widely used drying methods involve exposing food to heated air. Forced-air drying is used largely with grains, fruits, and vegetables. The so-called atmospheric batch-driers, such as kilns, are generally used when the drying operation is small or seasonal. Atmospheric-drying, in which the food moves through tunnels on a conveyer belt while the air flow is carefully controlled, is a technique commonly employed when the drying operation is more or less continuous.

Other methods of drying foods expose the product to a heated surface in a revolving drum. In this conductive drying method, the equipment may operate at atmospheric pressure or in a vacuum, which accelerates drying. Certain liquids (e.g., milk) can be spray-dried to produce powders suitable for later dissolution. Spray-drying can be effective for liquid foods that are especially vulnerable to heat and oxidation.

In the method known as freeze-drying, water is removed from foods by changing it from a solid (ice) to a gaseous state (water vapour), without permitting it to pass through the intermediate liquid phase, a transformation known as sublimation. Freeze-drying is carried out in a vacuum and at very low temperatures. It produces the best results of any drying method, principally because the food does not suffer significant loss of flavour or nutritional value. The process is expensive, however, because it requires both low and high temperatures and vacuum conditions. Its use seems justified only when the food being processed is very heat-sensitive and the resulting product must meet the highest possible standards of quality.

Suitable packaging is required for a great number of dehydrated foods to ensure satisfactory shelf life and to minimize losses due to water absorption and oxidation, as well as insect infestation.

Heat treatment

Cooking of food is such a ubiquitous and ancient practice that its role in food preservation is easily overlooked. Yet various forms of heat treatment — baking, broiling, roasting, boiling, frying, and stewing — are among the most widely used food processing techniques, in industry as well as in the home. Heat not only produces desirable changes in food, but can also lengthen safe storage times. Heating reduces the number of organisms and destroys some life-threatening microbial toxins. It inactivates enzymes that contribute to spoilage, makes foods more digestible, alters texture, and enhances flavour. But heating can also produce unwanted results, including loss of nutrients and adverse changes in flavour and aroma.

The temperature and length of time involved are critical in heat processing, especially when heat is being used to destroy microorganisms. A major goal of thermal processing is to achieve maximum destruction of organisms with minimum loss of food quality. This balance is often struck by the use of high temperatures for a comparatively short time.

As a method for reducing the number of microorganisms, heat treatment of food consists primarily of blanching, pasteurization, and sterilization. Blanching, exposing food briefly to hot water or steam, is normally used before foods are further processed by freezing, drying, or canning. In addition to cleansing the raw food product, blanching reduces the microbial load, removes accumulated gases, and inactivates enzymes. In the industrial setting, problems associated with food blanching, and with pasteurization or sterilization, include the disposal of large amounts of waste water, the unintended removal of solids from the food, damage to heat-sensitive products, and energy conservation.

The heat tolerance of microorganisms is influenced by acidity. Therefore, the temperature at which foods are canned depends on the acidity of the food being processed. Low-acid foods must be heated to high temperatures, under pressure, in specially designed pressure vessels (retorts) to ensure that hazardous microorganisms are effectively controlled. Acid foods, or foods that contain low levels of preservatives, can be processed at lower temperatures. Depending on the product and process employed the food may be packaged before or after heat treatment.

In the heat treatment of low-acid foods by sterilization, the objective is what is termed "commercial sterility", and the most important goal is destruction of spores of the bacterium *Clostridium botulinum*. A toxin produced by this organism is the cause of botulism, one of the most lethal forms of foodborne disease.

Some low-acid foods are also processed at lower temperatures in order to destroy pathogenic microorganisms and extend their shelf-life. This process is usually referred to as "pasteurization". The resulting product is not always stable indefinitely, and unless the distribution system can ensure that the product can be distributed rapidly to the consumer, or else kept at adequately low temperatures, the product may deteriorate quickly. The range of products treated in this way is quite large, and the conditions of treatment and distribution vary considerably. Pasteurization can be applied to milk, beer, and fruit juices, and even to some solid products such as canned meats.

The health protection benefits of heat treatment are lost, of course, if the food is not packaged in a way that protects it against subsequent contamination. Thermally processed products are normally packed in metal (e.g., tinplate, aluminium), glass or laminated plastic containers. Aseptic packaging of foods is a relatively new technique, in which the unpackaged product is heated quickly to a sterilization temperature, held there until sterile, aseptically cooled and poured into sterilized containers, which are then sealed.

The facilities and equipment necessary to ensure proper handling and packaging of processed foods are complex. As is the case with all modern food processing, these facilities require constant surveillance by trained personnel and frequent inspection by public health authorities responsible for the enforcement of food safety regulations.

If properly processed and packaged, heat-treated foods are microbially stable for long periods. Shelf-life is limited only by the slow physical and chemical changes caused by the interaction of contents and packaging and by the conditions in which the packaged food is stored.

Freezing

Freezing is the best method now in general use for the long-term preservation of food. Frozen food retains most of its original flavour, colour, and nutritive value. Despite its superiority, however, freezing often produces detrimental effects on food texture as a result of ice formation. Fast freezing minimizes this problem.

Preservation by freezing is achieved by lowering the temperature of the food to at least $-18°C$, which crystallizes all the water in the product to ice. At these low temperatures, microbial growth ceases and destructive enzyme activity, while not completely stopped, is reduced to an acceptable level. With some foods, such as vegetables, where enzyme activity during storage or thawing is critical, heat treatment, or some other means of destroying enzymes, is carried out prior to freezing. Food can be frozen before or after packaging.

Unpackaged foods freeze faster but are subject to considerable water loss unless they are frozen very rapidly.

Initially, the practice was to freeze food by placing it in a cold room ($-18°C$ to $-40°C$) and allowing air to circulate slowly over the food — a technique known as sharp-freezing. Later, air-blast freezers were developed for both batch and continuous processing. Their use has significantly reduced processing time and improved the quality of frozen products.

Food can also be frozen by being placed between, and in direct contact with, two hollow metal surfaces that are cooled by chilled brine or vaporizing refrigerants (ammonia or freon). This method, called plate-freezing, is slower than freezing in circulating air, but it minimizes dehydration. The food product must be packaged before it is processed by plate-freezing. In the process called cryogenic freezing, the product, usually unpackaged, is exposed to an extremely cold refrigerant that is undergoing a change of phase, e.g., from liquid to gas. The refrigerants most commonly used in the food industry are liquid nitrogen and liquid carbon dioxide. This method affords very fast freezing; hence damage to the product is kept to a minimum.

Obviously, frozen food must be maintained at or below freezing temperatures at all times if this method of preservation is to be effective. In addition, frozen food must be packed in containers that prevent moisture loss and oxidation, i.e., freezer burn. While the overall costs of thermal treatment and freezing are similar up to the completion of the processing operation, the need for an unbroken chain of transportation and storage at freezing temperatures places serious economic constraints on the use of freezing for the preservation of food.

Each method used to control spoilage and deterioration of food and to protect the consumer against foodborne disease has both advantages and disadvantages. Research is being undertaken, however, in many countries to make all these methods more effective and efficient.

Chapter 2

THE PROCESS OF FOOD IRRADIATION

Irradiation has the same objectives as other food processing methods — the reduction of losses due to spoilage and deterioration and control of the microbes and other organisms that cause foodborne diseases. But the techniques and equipment employed to irradiate food, the health and safety requirements that have to be taken into account, and a variety of problems that are unique to this way of processing food, put food irradiation into a category by itself. An understanding of how irradiation compares with the more conventional ways of processing food should begin with a brief, non-technical account of what the process is and how it works.

Ionizing radiation

Many of the traditional methods of food processing make use of energy in one form or another — the heat used in canning and sun-drying, for example. Food irradiation employs a particular form of electromagnetic energy, the energy of ionizing radiation. X-rays, which are a form of ionizing radiation, were discovered in 1895. Radioactivity and its associated ionizing radiations, alpha, beta, and gamma rays, were discovered the following year. (The term "ionizing radiation" has been used to describe these various rays because they cause whatever material they strike to produce electrically charged particles, called ions.)

Early experiments showed that ionizing radiation kills bacteria. There followed a number of isolated efforts to use this newly discovered energy to destroy the bacteria responsible for food spoilage. Promising and scientifically interesting as they were, these early efforts did not lead to the use of ionizing radiation by the food industry. At the turn of the century and for many years thereafter, there was no cost-effective way of obtaining radiation sources in the quantity required for industrial application. The X-ray generators of the day were very inefficient in converting electric power to X-rays, and the naturally occurring radioactive materials, such as radium, were too scarce to provide gamma rays, or other forms of radiation, in sufficient quantities for food processing.

In the early 1940s, advances in two areas paved the way for the economic production of sources of ionizing radiation in the amounts needed for industrial food processing. Machines, principally electron accelerators, were designed and developed that could generate ionizing radiation in unprecedented amounts and at acceptable cost. The other avenue of discovery was the study of atomic fission, which produced not only nuclear energy, but also fission products, such as caesium-137, that were themselves sources of ionizing radiation. The related discovery that certain elements could be made radioactive led to the production of other gamma-ray sources, such as cobalt-60. These advances stimulated renewed interest in food irradiation. Investigations using these new energy sources made it increasingly evident that ionizing radiation had the potential, at least, to become a powerful weapon in the battle against preventable food loss and foodborne illness.

Uses of food irradiation

Many of the practical applications of food irradiation have to do with preservation. Radiation inactivates food spoilage organisms, including bacteria, moulds, and yeasts. It is effective in lengthening the shelf-life of fresh fruits and vegetables by controlling the normal biological changes associated with ripening, maturation, sprouting, and finally aging. For example, radiation delays the ripening of green bananas, inhibits the sprouting of potatoes and onions, and prevents the greening of endive and white potatoes. Radiation also destroys disease-causing organisms, including parasitic worms and insect pests, that damage food in storage. As with other forms of food processing, radiation produces some useful chemical changes in food. For example, it softens legumes (beans), and thus shortens the cooking time. It also increases the yield of juice from grapes, and speeds the drying rate of plums.

Studies carried out since the 1940s demonstrating the benefits of food irradiation have also identified its limitations and some problems. For example, because radiation tends to soften some foods, especially fruit, the amount (or dose) of radiation that can be used is limited. Also, some irradiated foods develop an undesirable flavour. This problem can be avoided in meats if they are irradiated while frozen. However, no satisfactory method has yet been found to prevent the development of an off-flavour in irradiated dairy products. In some foods, the flavour problem can be prevented by using smaller amounts of radiation. The small amount of radiation required to control *Trichinella spiralis* in pork, for example, does not change the flavour of the meat.

Radiation dose

The radiation dose — the quantity of radiation energy absorbed by the food — is the most critical factor in food irradiation. Often, for each different kind of food, a specific dose has to be delivered to achieve a desired result. If the amount of radiation delivered is less than the appropriate dose, the intended effect may not be achieved. Conversely, if the dose is excessive, the food product may be so damaged as to be rendered unacceptable.

The special name for the unit of absorbed dose is the gray (Gy). It is defined as the mean energy imparted by ionizing radiation to matter per unit mass. One Gy is equal to one joule per kilogram. (An older unit of radiation measurement, the rad, equals 0.01 Gy). At present, the dose of radiation recommended by the FAO/WHO Codex Alimentarius Commission for use in food irradiation does not exceed 10 000 grays, usually written 10 kGy. This is actually a very small amount of energy, equal to the amount of heat required to raise the temperature of water by 2.4°C. With this small amount of energy, it is not surprising that food is little altered by the irradiation process, or that food receiving this amount of radiation is considered safe for human consumption.

Sources of ionizing radiation

As has been mentioned, an essential requirement for the industrial use of food irradiation is an economic source of radiation energy. Two types of radiation source can satisfy this requirement today: machines and man-made materials. Although they differ in the method of operation, both types of source produce identical effects on foods, microorganisms, and insects.

Machines called electron accelerators produce electron radiation, a form of ionizing radiation. Electrons are sub-atomic particles having very small mass and a negative electric charge. Beams of accelerated electrons can be used to irradiate foods at relatively low cost. This cost advantage is offset, however, by the fact that accelerated electron beams can penetrate food only to a maximum depth of about 8 cm, which is not deep enough to meet all the goals of food irradiation. Accelerated electrons are, therefore, particularly useful for treating grain or animal feed that can be processed in thin layers; electron beam irradiation is particularly suitable for these applications because of the very high throughputs involved in grain handling and the convenience of being able to switch the machine on and off at will.

Another machine source of ionizing radiation is the X-ray generator. An X-ray is a wave-form of energy similar to light. Unlike accelerated electrons, X-rays have great power to penetrate some materials. But as the early experimenters found, converting electricity into X-rays is a very inefficient, hence expensive, operation. The X-ray machines available for food processing have generally been adapted from those used in medical and industrial radiography and are not well suited to supply the power needed for food processing. Recent developments suggest that these problems of cost and power output may be solved by a new type of X-ray generator.

Man-made radionuclides constitute the other main source of ionizing radiation; radionuclides are radioactive materials that, as they decay, give off ionizing gamma-rays that can be used for food processing. One radionuclide that is readily available in large quantities is cobalt-60, which is produced by exposing naturally occurring cobalt-59 to neutrons in a nuclear reactor. The availability of another radionuclide, caesium-137, a by-product of nuclear reactor operations, is limited and it is not used widely at present. Gamma-rays from either of these radionuclides will penetrate deeply enough to meet virtually all food irradiation needs. The cost of man-made radionuclide sources is considered acceptable for industrial food irradiation in view of the great versatility and penetrating capacity of the gamma-rays.

The process

During the irradiation process food is exposed to the energy source in such a way that a precise and specific dose is absorbed. To do that it is necessary to know the energy output of the source per unit of time, to have a defined spatial relationship between the source and the target, and to expose the target material for a specific time. The radiation dose ordinarily used in food processing ranges from 50 Gy to 10 kGy and depends on the kind of food being processed and the desired effect.

Food irradiation plants vary as regards design and physical arrangement according to the intended use, but essentially there are two types: batch and continuous. In a batch facility, a given quantity of food is irradiated for a precise period of time. The cell in which food is irradiated is then unloaded and another batch is loaded and irradiated. In continuous irradiation facilities, food is passed through the cell at a controlled rate calculated to ensure that all the food receives exactly the intended dose.

Batch facilities are simpler to design and operate than continuous facilities and are more flexible. A wide range of dosages can be employed and they are well adapted to experimentation. Continuous facilities, on the other hand, are better able to accommodate large volumes of the product, especially when treating a single food at a given dose. Continuous operations are usually preferred in the food industry, partly because they offer a significant economy of scale.

Both machine and radionuclide energy sources must be installed in a shielded cell specially designed to prevent exposure of personnel to radiation. A machine source is simpler to operate because it can be turned off when personnel need to enter the cell to load the product or to carry out servicing and maintenance. With a radionuclide source, radiation is produced continuously; there is no way to turn it off. It is necessary, therefore, to provide a separate shielded storage space into which the source can be withdrawn when personnel have to enter the cell. Usually this consists of a pool of water deep enough to provide shielding from the gamma-rays when the radiation source is submerged.

With both machine sources and radionuclides, controls outside the cell guide and monitor the operation of the plant — they control the movement of the source from the storage to the operating position and vice versa (or turn on and off a radiation-generating machine) and control the operation of the food transport system that carries the food material into and out of the cell in a continuous operation, or the timer in a batch system.

The path taken by food in a continuous irradiation operation is usually fixed (see Fig. 1). It may be a simple, single-pass system or one whose pattern is more elaborate, providing exposure of the food

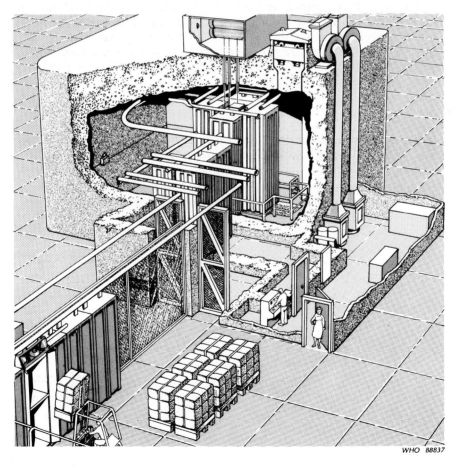

Fig. 1. Schematic diagram showing layout of a continuous facility for food irradiation.

to the radiation source from more than one direction. These more sophisticated systems are sometimes employed to achieve a more uniform dose and to make more efficient use of the radiation source. Since the energy output of a radionuclide source cannot be changed and the spatial relationship between source and target is fixed, the one variable commonly used to control dosage is exposure time, which can be adjusted as needed by regulating the speed of the transport mechanism. Obviously the dose absorbed will decrease as the speed of the transport mechanism is increased and vice versa.

Most food irradiation plants operate at a fixed location. There are, however, circumstances in which a mobile irradiator is useful. For example, foods produced seasonally may be available for processing in a given region only for a limited time. In such cases, it may be advantageous to move the irradiator to the product rather than the product to the facility. Moreover, there can be instances in which a mobile irradiator offers the means of improving the effectiveness of irradiation. With certain seafoods, for instance, irradiation should be carried out as soon as possible after the catch. If other factors dictate a long interval between harvest and processing, an on-site, mobile facility may offer the best approach to processing the product.

Costs

The cost of irradiating food has been estimated at between US$0.02 and US$ 0.40 per kilogram. This wide range results from the many variables involved in any one irradiation operation. Among them are the dose of radiation employed (which can vary widely depending on the purpose of the treatment), the volume and type of product being irradiated, the type and efficiency of the radiation source, whether the facility handles one or a variety of food products, the cost of transporting food to and from the irradiator, special packaging of the food, and the cost of supplementary processing such as freezing or heating. Construction of an irradiation plant large enough to permit economic operation has been estimated to cost in the order of several million US dollars.

The existing limited industrial experience with food irradiation makes it difficult to assess how the costs of this process might compare with those of other food processing technologies. It seems reasonably certain, however, from knowledge gained through research and development as well as practical application, that the benefits of food irradiation make its costs competitive.

Chapter 3

EFFECTS OF FOOD IRRADIATION

All decisions about the acceptability of irradiated food, whether they are personal choices by consumers or policy decisions by governments, reflect an assessment of the effects that irradiation has on the food itself, on the organisms and other matter that may contaminate the food, and most important, on the health and wellbeing of the consumers. Unless the benefits of irradiation clearly outweigh its disadvantages, irradiated food does not merit approval. And certainly, even the greatest technical benefits could not justify approval if there were unresolved doubts about the safety of irradiated food.

This chapter summarizes the results of numerous studies of the effects of irradiation, and presents the judgements on the safety of food irradiation reached by various international organizations and groups of experts.

Induced radioactivity

At high energy levels, ionizing radiation can make certain constituents of the food radioactive. Below a certain threshold of energy, however, these reactions do not occur. On the basis of experimental studies and theoretical estimates, in 1980, the Joint FAO/IAEA/WHO Expert Committee on the Wholesomeness of Irradiated Foods recommended restricting the radiation sources used in food processing to those with energy levels well below those that induce radioactivity in treated food.[1] Food processed by radiation in accordance with the Committee's recommendations does not become radioactive. However, the chemical composition of food can be altered by radiation, and authorities responsible for assessing the safety of irradiated food have had to consider the possibility that some of the chemical compounds formed during food irradiation may be harmful.

Animal studies

Extensive animal feeding studies designed to detect the presence of toxic substances in various irradiated foods have been carried out since the 1950s, mostly in the United States of America and the United Kingdom. In the mid-1960s, health authorities in both coun-

---
[1] WHO Technical Report Series, No. 659, 1981.

tries declared that food irradiated in accordance with established procedures was wholesome, which the Surgeon General of the United States Army defined as being safe and nutritionally adequate.

At about the same time, however, the US Food and Drug Administration (FDA) began to insist on more stringent evidence of safety. In 1968, the FDA withdrew approval of irradiated bacon. Evidence from animal feeding studies that had been deemed acceptable in 1963 when approval was granted was later judged by the FDA to be insufficient. The United States Army, which had originally sought approval to irradiate bacon, began a massive programme to test the safety of radiation-sterilized beef. Other countries also began to insist on further testing to clarify the safety of irradiated foods, and the volume and scope of research on irradiated foods rapidly expanded.

Animal feeding studies are costly. So, in 1970 FAO and IAEA, with advice from WHO, took the lead in creating the International Project in the Field of Food Irradiation. This project set out to bring uniformity to the various animal studies performed around the world in which animals were fed on food irradiated at or below 10 kGy; it helped to cut the cost of such studies and aided the exchange of information. Twenty-four countries participated in the project. Feeding studies were conducted with irradiated wheat flour, potatoes, rice, iced ocean fish, mangoes, spices, dried dates, and cocoa powder. This list of foodstuffs was drawn up as being representative of the major classes of foods, to reflect considerations relating to international trade, the importance of certain products in developing countries, and the suitability of the products for radiation treatment at doses up to 10 kGy. During its 12 years of existence, the project produced 67 technical reports, as well as numerous publications in scientific journals. Two extensive monographs were published in book form.

None of the studies carried out under the auspices of the project showed any indication that the irradiated foods contained radiation-produced carcinogens or other toxic substances. The project was terminated in 1982, having clearly established the wholesomeness of food irradiated at or below 10 kGy.

Many other studies were carried out by national research programmes during the 12 years that the project was under way. Several are of special importance because they differed from the usual procedure of feeding irradiated food to laboratory animals in order to assess carcinogenicity and other toxic effects. In a French study, for example, nine chemical coumpounds that had been identified in irradiated starch were fed daily to rats in amounts calculated to be 800 times the amounts the animals might be expected to consume from a normal daily intake of irradiated starch. No toxic effect was found even at this exaggerated rate of intake.

In most of the animal feeding studies carried out, irradiated foods comprised some 30% of the animals' daily food intake. However, in some studies, many generations of animals were raised on a diet consisting entirely of irradiated food, and no carcinogenic or other toxic effects were seen.

A recent American study of irradiated chicken meat is also significant, both because of the extent of the investigation and the high dose (58 kGy) of radiation involved. Dogs, mice and fruit flies were fed either electron-irradiated, gamma-irradiated, heat-sterilized, or enzyme-inactivated (blanched) chicken meat that had been stored frozen. No radiation-related adverse effects were observed, in spite of the fact that the meat was treated with a dose almost six times higher than that currently recommended for foods for human consumption.

While the great majority of animal feeding studies have demonstrated that irradiated foods have no harmful effects, the results of some studies have required careful re-evaluation. When animals on an irradiated test diet thrive better than control animals fed non-irradiated food it is normal to suspect a statistical error. But when animals on the test (irradiated) diet do less well than controls it is normal to suspect the diet not the statistics. Usually repeat studies do indeed disclose either faulty experimental design or incorrect evaluation of results. Sometimes they identify a biological variable that had not been taken into account. One investigator, for example, thought he had seen damage to the heart muscle of mice fed an irradiated diet. When the study was repeated with a much larger number of mice, the heart muscle lesion was not seen. In another study, rats on a diet that included 35% by weight of radiation-sterilized beef developed internal bleeding after long-term feeding. It was later shown that the level of vitamin K, a nutrient important in blood-clotting, was very low in this diet even before the inclusion of the irradiated beef, and that the further loss of vitamin K due to irradiation was enough to cause the bleeding. Adding vitamin K to the animals' diet eliminated the problem.

A study in which children were fed irradiated food is frequently cited to show that these foods are unsafe for human use. Malnourished Indian children who were fed freshly irradiated wheat for 4-6 weeks reportedly showed more chromosomal changes than children fed irradiated wheat that had been stored for 12 weeks prior to use. Several animal feeding studies conducted in the same country and elsewhere did not confirm this finding. An FAO/IAEA/WHO Expert Committee on the Wholesomeness of Irradiated Foods examined this issue in 1976 and concluded that the significance of the reported chromosomal changes was not clear, since the natural frequency of such changes is highly variable.[1] Subsequently, health agencies and expert committees in Denmark, the United Kingdom, and the United States of America concluded that the original Indian study did not demonstrate an adverse effect of irradiation. When human volunteers in China consumed various irradiated foods for periods of 7-15 weeks, they showed no signs of any adverse health effects, including chromosomal changes.

Chemical studies

If extensive animal feeding studies have established the safety of irradiated wheat, what do they imply about the safety of irradiated rye or rice? Do results obtained with unpackaged whole fish also apply to irradiated, vacuum-packed fish fillets? Obviously, an enormous number of lengthy and costly animal studies would be needed to answer every conceivable question about the safety of irradiation. In recent years, radiation chemistry has been recognized as an additional tool for toxicological evaluation, and the methods involved have been substantially refined. As a result, answers to questions about the safety of irradiated food can be extrapolated with reasonable confidence on the basis of information about the chemical composition of foods and the radiolytic effects (chemical changes caused by irradiation) produced under various conditions. An FAO/IAEA/WHO Expert Committee on the Wholesomeness of Irradiated Foods accepted this rationale in 1976, suggesting that the interpretation of radiolytic reactions would considerably reduce the need for conventional toxicological testing and would, moreover, greatly simplify the testing procedure.

Much is known about the substances formed when food is irradiated and the factors — such as temperature, humidity, and presence or absence of oxygen — that influence the formation of radiolytic products. The most important modifying factor, of course, is the radiation dose. For example, at the low dosages required for insect disinfestation of grain (less than 0.5 kGy), it is difficult to detect any chemical change in irradiated food. At high doses, such as those that would be required for sterilization (above 30 kGy), many chemical changes may occur.

Another interesting observation is that while individual food components, such as amino acids, vitamins, and sugars, can be destroyed by irradiation, they are invariably less susceptible to damage when irradiated in the complex, and evidently protective, matrix of an intact food product. Furthermore, radiolytic products are not very unusual, and they are not found uniquely in irradiated food. One study showed that beef treated with 60 kGy of radiation contained some 60 detectable radiolytic products. Most, however,

---
[1] WHO Technical Report Series, No. 604, 1977.

were produced in small amounts, and all were detectable also in various unirradiated food products.

The comparatively low yields of radiolytic products and the fact that none of them is unique to foods treated with radiation mean that there is at present no reliable method of identifying foods that have been irradiated at the dosages normally used in food processing.

Changes in sensory characteristics

The chemical changes that radiation produces in food may lead to noticeable effects on flavour. The extent of these effects depends principally on the type of food being irradiated, on the radiation dose, and on various other factors, such as temperature, during radiation processing.

Some foods react unfavourably even to low doses of radiation. Milk and certain other dairy products are among the most radiation-sensitive foods. Doses as low as 0.1 kGy will impart an off-flavour to milk that most consumers find unacceptable.

The high radiation dose required for sterilization has been associated with unwanted flavour changes in meat, and it appears that the change occurs in the lean rather than the fat portion of meat. Irradiation of lean cuts of meat produces more off-flavour than irradiation of cuts with a higher fat content. Furthermore, pork is less adversely affected than beef or veal, presumably because of its higher fat content. The off-flavour is most pronounced immediately after irradiation; it decreases or disappears during storage and cooking. Investigators have also observed that meat irradiated at low temperature is less liable to flavour change. Enzyme-inactivated, vacuum-packed beef, chicken, pork, and various meat products that received about 50 kGy of radiation at a temperature of $-30°C$ for long-term shelf-stability were judged to have an acceptable flavour by panels of food experts and consumers in one study.

Colour is another property of meat that can be changed by irradiation. Doses higher than 1.5 kGy may cause a brown discoloration of meat exposed to air.

The practical upper dosage limit for the irradiation of fruits and vegetables is determined by effects on the firmness of the plant tissue. Depending on the product being processed, radiation doses of 1-3 kGy will cause softening of some fruits. This effect is not really a direct result of the radiation; it is, instead, a physiological response — the breakdown of cell membranes by the action of enzymes. This softening is not immediately noticeable; it begins to appear hours or even days after the exposure to radiation.

Other sensory or physical changes caused by irradiation include a thinning (reduced viscosity) of soups and gravies whose starch components, such as potatoes and grains, have been irradiated. The effect is not seen at the relatively low doses required to inhibit sprouting or control insects, but it can occur at higher doses — above 1 kGy. In certain situations, this effect of irradiation is desirable. It appears to account for the reduced cooking time required for dry soups and also to improve the rehydration properties of dried fruits.

Changes in nutritional quality

Food processing and preparation methods in general tend to result in some loss of nutrients. As in other chemical reactions produced by irradiation, nutritional changes are primarily related to dose. The composition of the food and other factors, such as temperature and the presence or absence of air, also influence nutrient loss. At low doses, up to 1 kGy, the loss of nutrients from food is insignificant. In the medium-dose range, 1-10 kGy, some vitamin loss may occur in food exposed to air during irradiation or storage. At high dosages, 10-50 kGy, vitamin loss can be mitigated by protective measures — irradiation at low temperatures and exclusion of air during processing and storage. The use of these measures can hold the vitamin loss associated with high dosage to the levels seen with medium-range doses when protective measures are not employed.

Some vitamins — riboflavin, niacin, and vitamin D — are fairly insensitive to irradiation. Others, such as vitamins A, B_1, E, and K are more easily destroyed. Little is known about the effect of irradiation on folic acid, and conflicting results have been reported concerning the effects of irradiation on vitamin C in fruits and vegetables.

The significance of radiation-induced vitamin loss in a particular food depends, of course, on how important that food is as a source of vitamins for the people who consume it. For example, if a specific food product is the sole dietary source of vitamin A for a given population, then radiation processing of that particular food may be inadvisable because it could greatly reduce the availability of this essential nutrient. Furthermore, since many irradiated foods are cooked before use, the cumulative loss of vitamins through processing and cooking should be taken into account. Chemical analyses and animal feeding studies have shown that the nutritional value of proteins is little affected by irradiation, even at high doses. Animal studies in various species have also demonstrated that the effects of radiation on other nutrients are minimal.

Effects on microorganisms

Microorganisms (especially Gram-negative bacteria such as salmonellae) can be destroyed by irradiation. Bacterial spores, however, are killed only by high doses, which means that the highly lethal foodborne disease, botulism, is not necessarily prevented by irradiation.

A given radiation dose will kill a certain proportion of the microbial population exposed to it, regardless of the number of microorganisms present. This property, or result, of radiation treatment implies that the higher the pretreatment population of spoilage bacteria, for example, the higher the population will be after the food has been irradiated. And, of course, if spoilage has already begun, radiation can do nothing to reverse it. Consequently, as with any other method of food preservation, irradiation is not a substitute for good hygienic practice in food production and processing.

Exactly what portion of a given population of microorganisms will be destroyed by irradiation depends, as do many other radiation effects, on several factors, including the temperature at which the radiation treatment is carried out. Higher temperatures make organisms more sensitive to radiation; some microorganisms are more affected by radiation when the moisture content of food is high. At a given dose, microorganisms are less sensitive to radiation when incorporated in food than when suspended in water.

Apprehension persists that radiation processing of food might pose a public health hazard by causing radiation-resistant microbes to flourish, or by producing mutant strains of disease-causing microbes that neither food processing techniques nor the human immune system could control. The results of research to examine these potential risks have been reassuring. It appears that microorganisms surviving a dose of radiation are injured. They are more vulnerable to the destructive effects of storage in conditions (such as cold) that are unfavourable to microbial growth, and they are more likely to be killed by cooking. Nevertheless, pathogenic microorganisms that survive radiation treatment, like those that are not killed by heat processing or other measures, can pose a public health probem, not because radiation has in some way changed them but because they are still alive. Unless a sterilizing dose of radiation has been delivered, irradiated foods must be stored and handled with the same regard for safety as that accorded to non-irradiated or other unsterilized foods.

The judgement of international organizations and experts

The first international meeting devoted exclusively to a discussion of scientific data on the wholesomeness of irradiated foods and the legislative aspects of food irradiation was held in Brussels in 1961 under the sponsorship of FAO, IAEA, and WHO. The meeting was attended by representatives from 28 countries. Although the results of numerous long-term feeding studies were presented by delegates from several countries, the meeting concluded that it would be premature to authorize industrial food irradiation. The group recommended that the three sponsoring organizations should form a committee of experts to advise on the wholesomeness of radiation-processed foods. A Joint FAO/IAEA/WHO Expert Committee on the Technical Basis for Legislation on Irradiated Food, which was convened in response to that recommendation, held a meeting in Rome in 1964.

The Rome meeting was unequivocal in its conclusion about the safety of irradiated foods. Having reviewed feeding studies in animals and human volunteers, the Joint Committee concluded that "irradiated food treated in accordance with procedures that should be followed in approved practice, have given no indication of adverse effects of any kind, and there has been no evidence that the nutritional value of irradiated food is affected in any important way." The Committee endorsed the regulatory control of food irradiation, including the establishment of lists of foods for which irradiation would be permitted at specified doses, and the identification of tests to assess the safety for human consumption of individual food products treated by irradiation. It suggested that the tests should be broadly similar to those used to assess conventional food additives.

When a Joint FAO/IAEA/WHO Committee met next in Geneva in 1969, it granted temporary approval to potatoes irradiated at doses up to 0.15 kGy and wheat and wheat products treated at doses up to 0.75 kGy. The temporary nature of the approval meant that the Committee felt additional testing was needed to confirm the safety of these products. At the same meeting, the Committee concluded that it did not have enough data to reach a judgement on the safety of irradiated onions. At a meeting in Geneva in 1976, having reviewed the additional testing called for earlier, a Joint Committee gave unconditional approval to irradiated potatoes (up to 0.15 kGy), wheat (up to 1 kGy), papayas (up to 1 kGy), strawberries (up to 3 kGy), and chicken (up to 7 kGy). Provisional approval, which replaced the former temporary approval, was given to onions, rice, fresh cod, and redfish, meaning that the Committee wanted further tests to be carried out. It declined to rule on the safety of irradiated mushrooms, declaring the available data to be inadequate.

When a Joint Committee met in 1980 in Geneva, it was presented with a wealth of testing data, most of it generated by the International Project in the Field of Food Irradiation. Finally, having what it believed to be wholly sufficient and satisfactory scientific information, the Committee concluded that "the irradiation of any food commodity up to an overall average dose of 10 kGy presents no toxicological hazard; hence toxicological testing of foods so treated is no longer required." It also found that irradiation up to 10 kGy "introduces no special nutritional or microbiological problems."

At the request of FAO and WHO, the Board of the International Committee on Food Microbiology and Hygiene of the International Union of Microbiological Societies met in Copenhagen in 1982 to reconsider the evidence for the microbiological safety of the process. The Board found no cause for concern and endorsed the conclusions reached earlier by the Joint Committee. The Board concluded that food irradiation was an important addition to the methods of control of foodborne pathogens and did not present any additional hazards to health.

The Commission of the European Community asked its Scientific Committee on Food for advice on the wholesomeness of suitably irradiated foods. In 1986, the Scientific Committee essentially endorsed the findings and conclusions of the FAO/IAEA/WHO Joint Expert Committee and affirmed the view that further animal testing to ascertain the safety of irradiated foods was unnecessary.

Chapter 4

PRACTICAL APPLICATIONS OF FOOD IRRADIATION

Extensive research during the past four decades has documented the usefulness and safety of ionizing radiation as a food processing technique. But its potential value, of course, can be realized only if the technique is put to practical use. This chapter summarizes information on the practical application of irradiation in the processing of food — how it is used and with what results. The chapter concludes with a discussion of the special problems associated with irradiation of food in developing and developed countries, and especially in tropical regions.

Doses and effects of irradiation

For each application of food irradiation there is a minimum dose below which the intended effect will not be achieved. Table 1 shows the dose requirements for some typical uses of food irradiation.

Because irradiation causes only a slight temperature rise in the food being processed, it can kill microorganisms without thawing frozen food. Moreover, an effective radiation dose can be delivered through most standard food packaging materials, including those that cannot withstand heat. This means that irradiation can be applied to hermetically sealed products without the risk of recontamination or reinfestation of properly packaged foods.

Some food products may have to be irradiated under special conditions, for example at low temperature or in an oxygen-free atmosphere. Others, as noted previously, may undergo multiple processing, using, for example, both ionizing radiation and heat. This particular combination may allow the use of lower radiation doses because heat makes microorganisms more sensitive to the effects of radiation. Since radiation does not damage packaging materials designed to hold food during irradiation, multiple processing is facilitated and is more economical.

The actual dose of radiation employed in any food processing application represents a balance between the amount needed to produce a desired result and the amount the product can tolerate without suffering unwanted change. High radiation doses can cause organoleptic changes (off-flavours or changes in texture), especially in foods of animal origin, such as dairy products. In fresh fruits and vegetables, radiation may cause softening and increase the

Table 1. Dose requirement in various applications of food irradiation

Purpose	Dose (kGy)[a]	Products
Low dose (up to 1 kGy)		
(a) Inhibition of sprouting	0.05-0.15	Potatoes, onions, garlic, ginger-root, etc.
(b) Insect disinfestation and parasite disinfection	0.15-0.50	Cereals and pulses, fresh and dried fruits, dried fish and meat, fresh pork, etc.
(c) Delay of physiological process (e.g. ripening)	0.50-1.0	Fresh fruits and vegetables
Medium dose (1-10 kGy)		
(a) Extension of shelf-life	1.0-3.0	Fresh fish, strawberries, etc.
(b) Elimination of spoilage and pathogenic microorganisms	1.0-7.0	Fresh and frozen seafood, raw or frozen poultry and meat, etc.
(c) Improving technological properties of food	2.0-7.0	Grapes (increasing juice yield), dehydrated vegetables (reduced cooking time), etc.
High dose (10-50 kGy)[b]		
(a) Industrial sterilization (in combination with mild heat)	30-50	Meat, poultry, seafood, prepared foods, sterilized hospital diets
(b) Decontamination of certain food additives and ingredients	10-50	Spices, enzyme preparations, natural gum, etc.

[a] Gy: gray - unit used to measure absorbed dose. For definition, see page 20

[b] Only used for special purposes. The Joint FAO/WHO Codex Alimentarius Commission has not yet endorsed high-dose applications (see Annex 2).

permeability of tissue. These effects may limit the permissible dose because they are often accompanied by accelerated spoilage if the product becomes contaminated by microorganisms after irradiation treatment. On the other hand, since irradiation slows the rate of ripening of fresh fruits and vegetables, properly stored and/or packaged products remain in a usable condition considerably longer than they would without radiation processing. The extent of radiation-induced organoleptic changes in fruits and vegetables is dose-related: there seems to be a threshold dose below which these changes are not detectable. For that reason, the selection of dosage and, often, the decision to employ supplementary processing to contribute to the intended result are critical factors. The environmental conditions may also strongly affect the dose response of the product from both textural and organoleptic aspects.

Some typical applications of food irradiation

Some examples of the use of radiation to enhance the safety and quality of food are explained below: these illustrations are representative of actual applications now being carried out industrially or experimentally in various countries.

Control of sprouting and germination

Radiation treatment at low doses inhibits the sprouting of potatoes and yam tubers, onions and garlic, ginger, and chestnuts. The dose required to inhibit sprouting of potatoes and yams is 0.08-0.14 kGy; for ginger it is 0.04-0.10 kGy; for onions, shallots, and garlic, 0.03-0.12 kGy; and for chestnuts, approximately 0.20 kGy. The appropriate dose within these ranges depends on the variety and other properties of the product.

Although, with some varieties, cooking darkens irradiated potatoes more than non-irradiated, and although irradiated potatoes are less resistant to rotting, commercial irradiation has been carried out since 1973 in Japan, where chemical sprout inhibitors are banned. The success of the Japanese system is due in large measure to careful handling of the product before and after treatment, including careful sorting, curing, and storage.

Irradiation is useful for the long-term inhibition of sprouting and preservation of the desirable qualities of onions and garlic during storage. Industrial irradiation of these products is being employed in the German Democratic Republic and Hungary. In other countries — Argentina, Bangladesh, Chile, Israel, the Philippines, Thailand, and Uruguay — pilot quantities of irradiated potatoes, onions, and garlic have been sold.

Controlling the germination of barley during malting is of considerable economic importance. Doses of 0.25-0.50 kGy applied to air-dried barley do not prevent the emergence of shoot tips and tendrils during malting, but markedly retard root growth. In this way, high quality malt can be obtained while the losses resulting from root growth are reduced. Since this effect of radiation processing persists for at least seven months, treatment can be applied before the barley is put into storage, with the added benefit of destroying any insect pests that may be present in the grain.

Very small radiation doses (0.01-0.10 kGy) stimulate the germination of barley, a result that can be used to shorten the malting process and increase the production capacity of malting plants.

Food irradiation

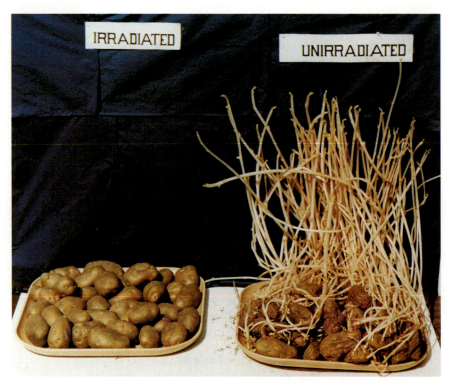

Fig. 2. Comparison of irradiated potatoes with untreated potatoes after 6 months of storage.

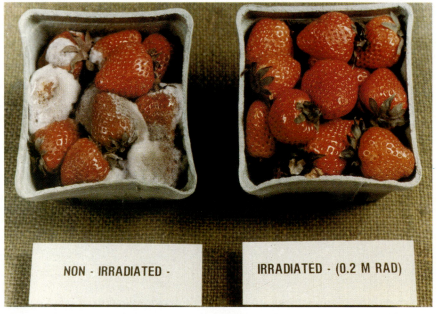

Fig. 3. Comparison of irradiated strawberries with untreated strawberries after 15 days of storage.

Practical applications

Insect disinfestation

Radiation at relatively low doses (up to 0.50 kGy) kills or sterilizes all the developmental stages of the common insect pests of grain, including eggs deposited inside the grain.

Dried fruits, vegetables, and nuts are liable to insect attack, and some of these products, especially fruits, cannot be effectively disinfested by either chemical or physical means other than irradiation. Application of 0.2-0.7 kGy to products that have been suitably packaged to prevent reinfestation eliminates the insect problem in dried fruits and vegetables and in nuts. The same technique could sharply reduce losses of dried fish, an important source of protein in many developing countries.

Radiation disinfestation can contribute significantly to improving trade in certain tropical and subtropical fruits, such as citrus fruit, mangoes, and papayas. Because it affords a residue-free means of preventing the importation of harmful insects, radiation treatment offers a viable alternative to fumigation to satisfy the quarantine regulations in a number of countries. Fruit flies, for example, and even the weevil that lodges deep inside the seed of the mango can be controlled by irradiation.

Radiation disinfestation is being performed on an industrial scale in the Soviet Union, where an electron irradiation plant to treat imported grains went into operation in 1980 at Port Odessa.

Shelf-life extension of perishable foods

One of the principal uses of food irradiation is for killing the microorganisms that cause spoilage or deterioration of the product. The amount of radiation needed to control or eliminate these organisms depends on the radiation tolerance of the particular organism and the number or "load" of such organisms in the particular volume of food to be treated.

The shelf-life of many fruits and vegetables, meat, poultry, and fish and other seafoods can be considerably prolonged — certainly doubled — by treatment with combinations of refrigeration and relatively low doses of radiation that do not alter flavour or texture. Most food spoilage microorganisms are killed at doses of less than 5 kGy. Various fresh fruits, including strawberries, mangoes, and papayas, have been irradiated and marketed successfully. A combination of mild heat treatment (immersion in hot water), low-dose irradiation, and proper packaging may be successfully applied to fruits that are sensitive to higher radiation doses.

Delaying ripening and aging of fruits and vegetables

Exposure to a low dose of radiation delays the ripening and/or senescence of some fruits and vegetables, thereby extending their shelf-life. This effect of radiation treatment was discovered in the course of studies of the role of radiation in controlling microorganisms. The magnitude and even the direction of such changes depend on the size of the dose and the state of ripeness at the time of treatment. A measurable extension of shelf-life may be obtained with doses of 0.3-1.0 kGy. This level of exposure will increase the shelf-life of mangoes by about one week and that of bananas by up to two weeks. Maturation of mushrooms and asparagus after harvesting can be retarded with doses in the range of 1.0-1.5 kGy.

Destruction of parasites

Irradiation inactivates certain parasitic organisms that are responsible for both human and animal diseases. The parasitic roundworm *Trichinella spiralis*, which causes trichinosis and is found in pork, is inactivated by radiation at a minimum dose of 0.15 kGy. Other parasites, including pork and beef tapeworms, the protozoon in pork responsible for toxoplasmosis, and various flukes that infest fish are rendered non-infective by low-dose radiation treatment.

Control of foodborne diseases

Foodborne illness caused by microorganisms is a major and increasing problem for the food processing and food service industries. For this reason, an important potential application of food irradiation is for decontamination to control foodborne disease. Radiation could play an equally important role in the processing of solid foods of animal origin and dry foods as does heat treatment (pasteurization) in the processing of fluid milk and fruit juices.

The relatively low dose of radiation needed to destroy non-spore-forming pathogenic bacteria in food, such as *Salmonella, Campylobacter, Listeria* and *Yersinia* can be very useful in controlling the serious public health problems caused by these organisms.

Extensive experience has demonstrated that radiation treatment under normal industrial conditions, at a dose that does not produce unacceptable changes in the food product, will eliminate pathogenic non-sporing bacteria in red meat, poultry, and fish. While all these food products are distributed both fresh and frozen, it appears that in some countries irradiation of frozen commodities is more feasible. A dose of 2-7 kGy is sufficient to control foodborne pathogens in frozen meats, poultry, egg pulp, shrimp, and frog legs without causing unacceptable changes in the product.

Irradiation is beneficial in controlling the microbial contamination of dry food ingredients, and this improves the safety and storage properties of foods prepared with them. Spices, dry vegetable seasonings, herbs, starch, protein concentrates, and commercial enzyme preparations used in the food industry are very often heavily contaminated with spoilage and pathogenic organisms, and can be decontaminated with radiation doses of 3-10 kGy with no adverse effects on their flavour, texture, or other properties. Microorganisms that survive this treatment are more susceptible to subsequent processing.

Radiation decontamination is becoming more widely used in several countries. Considerable amounts of frozen shrimps, prawns, and frog legs are irradiated in Belgium and the Netherlands at dose levels up to 4 kGy. Electron beam irradiation of blocks of mechanically deboned, frozen poultry products is carried out industrially in France. Large-scale gamma irradiation of fresh poultry has been evaluated in Canada. Increasing amounts of dry food ingredients are being irradiated in Belgium and the Netherlands. Spices are being irradiated in Argentina, Brazil, Denmark, Finland, France, Hungary, Israel, Norway, the United States of America and Yugoslavia.

In some countries, the packaging material used for long-life milk and milk products, as well as for fruit juices, is being sterilized by gamma-rays at doses between 15 and 25 kGy.

In a related application, radiation sterilization of meals prepared for hospitalized patients whose immune systems have been suppressed by disease or therapy has been approved in the Federal Republic of Germany, the Netherlands, and the United Kingdom. The variety, palatability, and nutritional quality of meals for these patients can apparently be improved if radiation sterilization is used in place of thermal sterilization. It seems reasonable that this application may prove useful among other population groups, such as air travellers and the young and old residents of nursing facilities.

Food preservation problems in tropical countries

The warm and humid climate and abundant rainfall found in many tropical countries combine to make them especially well suited to the use of irradiation as a means of food processing. Highly perishable foods, such as roots and tubers, fruits, vegetables, and fish, form the traditional diet of large tropical populations, while cereal grains and legumes are consumed in significant quantities. The major agricultural exports of tropical countries include coffee, cocoa, tea, spices, and sea products, together with an increasingly wide variety of fruits and vegetables. All these products can be effectively processed by irradiation.

Both the climate and the patterns of food production in tropical countries contribute to major post-harvest problems. The abundance of produce during and immediately after harvest creates storage problems that often result in food losses, because the physical and environmental conditions in centres of food production are often unfavourable for effective long-term storage. And finally, both the nature of the crops produced and the high temperature and humidity of tropical areas favour the rapid growth of spoilage organisms and accelerate chemical and physical deterioration of fruit and vegetable crops and seafood. For tropical grains, significant losses result from insect infestation, moulds, and premature germination. For tuber crops and onions, sprouting and attack by bacteria and fungi are the major causes of loss.

Insect infestation and contamination by fungi are especially serious problems in the tropics and result in not only serious food loss but also illness. At a temperature of about 32°C, a colony of 50 insects can multiply to 312 million in four months. Such a population in stored grain would result in enormous food loss.

Destruction caused by fungal attack is more commonly seen in warm, humid environments. It is therefore more serious in tropical coastal areas where a season of high humidity coincides with the period of food storage. The major problem caused by certain fungi is the development of toxins that may cause illness. Crops that have been damaged by moulds are often used as animal feed because of their inferior quality. As a result, human beings can be exposed to harmful toxins from both the contaminated grain and the animals fed on the grain. The toxic products of certain moulds, especially aflatoxin, have been shown to be powerful carcinogenic agents in certain animals, and they may have the same effect in man.

The economic impact of disease, including the loss of productivity associated with the consumption of unsafe food in tropical countries, is incalculable. But it is only a fraction of the total cost of food loss in those regions of the world. A survey in 1980 in the WHO African Region indicated that at least 20% of total food production was lost after harvest. Even at 1980 levels of production, a 50% reduction in the losses would annually save food to the value of US$ 1 800 million in the Region.

Food irradiation in developing countries: needs and problems

The scope of the agriculture- and food-related issues confronting developing nations is too broad to be addressed in this discussion. It should be noted, however, that many developing countries have set themselves the goal of self-sufficiency as regards food, and that for many others the export of food commodities is a major and essential source of income. For these reasons, the need to reduce food losses in developing countries is paramount. But it is no less important to prevent or control the causes of foodborne disease, both as a domestic public health goal and as an aid to successful international trade in foodstuffs.

Food irradiation, apart from reducing food losses and the risk of foodborne disease, may also offer special advantages over conventional food processing techniques in developing countries. For example, because many food preparations in developing countries are derived from fresh foods, the extension of the shelf-life of perishable foods by radiation treatment would increase the opportunities for marketing and distribution. However, developing countries will not be prepared to make the sizeable investments required to set up irradiation plants until the developed countries that import food give their approval to marketing food treated in this way.

In addition, a number of issues will have to be addressed before food irradiation can be successfully introduced in developing countries. Food irradiation requires not only highly trained personnel and specialized equipment, but also a regulatory system to ensure that the process will be carried out correctly. Many developing countries have not yet established the legislative and regulatory mechanisms and safety standards that will be required.

FAO, IAEA, and WHO have made information available to countries that provides a basis for the development of general operational and safety standards for food irradiation practices, and on the effect of irradiation on products as they are normally produced and handled in developing countries. This kind of information is obtained from pilot projects designed to establish irradiation dose ranges and to assess the effect of extending the shelf-life on the nutritional status of foods from developing countries. The results obtained in different studies may be expected to differ for different kinds of food, different methods of handling food products, and different environmental conditions, such as temperature and humidity.

Food irradiation is economically feasible only when there is a fairly large quantity of produce to be processed. In many developing countries, however, agricultural production is decentralized and transportation systems cannot bring foodstuffs together rapidly enough to make radiation processing practicable. Under such circumstances, small-scale, mobile, multipurpose irradiation facilities would seem most suitable. However, mobile irradiation facilities require constant checks in order to maintain the required safety levels. Such plants are at present only in the developmental stage. In countries that have a well established food export industry, of course, full-scale irradiation facilities could be located at the dockside or at air terminals.

Food irradiation requires facilities in addition to the processing plant itself. Specialized laboratories are needed to perform dosimetry tests to ensure that safety standards and quality control requirements are being met; and once the treatment has been applied a basic infrastructure must ensure that irradiated foods are properly handled, packaged, and stored (including cold storage). Cold storage requirements can impose major energy demands on countries in which the supply of readily available energy is severely restricted.

Investment will also be required to train the specialized manpower required for effective application of radiation food processing. Until the necessary training can be provided in the home country, these needs may have to be met by sending personnel abroad for training or by importing skilled manpower. Both approaches can be costly.

Most developing countries will probably need to import much of the equipment required for food irradiation. Contemporary designs of food irradiation plants are often more suited to the conditions and needs of developed countries. Designs that keep capital costs to a minimum and make the most effective use of relatively low-cost labour will be more suitable for developing countries, and such designs are already available.

Few studies have been conducted, however, on the economic feasibility of food irradiation in developing countries. Estimates made in 1982 suggested that costs would range from US$ 40 to US$ 70 per ton of fish. An FAO/IAEA group that examined the use of irradiation as a quarantine treatment for agricultural commodities estimated that disinfestation of fruits would cost less than US$ 60 and perhaps as little as US$ 20 per ton. It is clear, however, that more detailed and up-to-date information will be needed as regards costs to enable developing countries to gauge the applicability of irradiation to their produce and their situations.

Food irradiation in developed countries

In contrast to the situation in developing countries, the major food problems in developed countries concern microbial contamination of foods of animal origin — fish and shellfish, poultry, and red meat. Highly developed food processing and distribution systems, the wide availability of refrigeration throughout the distribution chain (as well as in homes), and the generally high standards of hygiene in developed countries make food spoilage a less pressing problem. Hence, the prevention of foodborne disease caused by both domestic and imported food products is the primary objective of food preservation measures in the developed world.

A significant proportion of the food consumed in developed countries is produced by large industries that serve caterers, retail food stores and supermarkets, and public and private institutions such as schools and hospitals. Some of the products of these industries are distributed all over the world. Under these conditions, outbreaks of foodborne disease originating from a single source can rapidly cause serious health problems of very broad scope. While disease outbreaks involving hundreds or thousands of people and numerous deaths, sometimes in several countries at once, receive wide media attention, it is undoubtedly true that many more instances of foodborne disease are largely unnoticed by the general public.

It is generally accepted that it is at present impossible to guarantee the production of raw foods of animal origin, particularly poultry and pork, without the presence of certain pathogenic microorganisms and parasites such as *Salmonella, Campylobacter, Listeria, Toxoplasma,* and *Trichinella.* These foods may pose a significant threat to public health.

As a consequence, processing by irradiation, either alone or in combination with other treatments, offers some unique advantages over conventional methods. They are:

(*a*) the opportunity to treat foods after packaging to prevent microbes in untreated foods from contaminating food that has already been processed;

(*b*) the conservation of food in the fresh state for long periods with no noticeable loss of quality, and;

(*c*) the economic savings from the use of a low-energy, low-cost processing technique when compared with other food processing methods, such as heat or refrigeration.

Irradiation could be of enormous value in dealing with the major food problems of developed countries. Yet despite endorsement by FAO and WHO and in particular by the Joint FAO/WHO Codex Alimentarius Commission, developed countries have been slow to adopt this technology; it is clear that one of the main reasons for this is the attitude of the public towards a technique involving radiation treatments. This is a problem that can only be tackled by public education.

Chapter 5

LEGISLATION AND CONTROL OF FOOD IRRADIATION

Every method of food processing results in some changes in the nature of the food that may have some consequences for consumers, but it is clear that irradiated food is wholesome and that its consumption, as part of the diet, is entirely without harmful effects.

As far as workers in the food industry are concerned, irradiation poses no greater risk than other technologies for food processing. Indeed, irradiation is safer than some food processing methods, such as those using hazardous substances, e.g., fumigants for the elimination of insects.

To ensure the necessary high degree of safety, governments need to enact regulations as regards both the irradiated food and the irradiation facilities. Regulatory agencies should determine which foods may be treated by irradiation and for what specific purposes, and should establish the precise amount of radiation that may be used in the processing of each type of food to achieve the desired effect. Regulatory agencies should also prescribe the type of information about the irradiation process that must be included in the labelling of irradiated foods. In this context, the Codex Alimentarius General Standard for the Labelling of Prepackaged Foods clearly states that a food that has been treated with ionizing radiation shall be labelled to indicate this fact. Food irradiation plants will be subject not only to the type of scrutiny given to all food processing operations, but also to regulation and oversight by government authorities responsible for the safety of other applications of irradiation. Thus, a dual system of control will ensure that food irradiation presents no undue risk to workers, consumers, or the environment.

Safety of the process

It is important to make it clear at the outset that the dose level used in food irradiation does not make the food, its packaging, or the equipment in the facility radioactive. Excessive radiation doses produce unacceptable changes in the taste, colour and texture of food. For this reason, food processors have a considerable incentive to ensure that the dose used to irradiate food is the minimum necessary to produce the intended result.

Dosimeters placed with the food product being irradiated measure the radiation to which it is exposed. This dosimetry information

Legislation and control

enables qualified plant personnel to monitor the process and to regulate the radiation dose. The operators can determine the most efficient arrangement of the product on the racks or conveyor belts and control other factors that influence the dose of radiation absorbed by the food.

Irradiation does not produce any discernible alteration of the food itself that can be used to verify that it has been irradiated or to measure the amount of absorbed radiation. Thus, there is, at present, no generally accepted, practical, scientific method for determining whether a food item has been irradiated; it is likely, however, that a technique to detect treated foods will be developed soon. At present the only way to know whether a food has been irradiated and how much radiation has been delivered during food processing is through detailed record-keeping and careful dose measurement during irradiation.

Radiation protection measures

Radiation protection activities are designed and regulated to prevent accidental irradiation of plant workers and the release of radiation into the environment. Although each of the 34 countries that has approved food irradiation has its own legislative approach to ensuring that such accidents do not occur, they all follow the broad pattern summarized below. (Readers seeking more detailed information should refer to the bibliography and the official regulations governing food irradiation in their own countries.)

Licensing

In addition to being licensed as food processing establishments, food irradiation plants should be licensed by the government agency responsible for the regulation of irradiation applications and installations. Such a licence should be granted only after a thorough investigation has established, among many other things, that the site for the plant is safe and appropriate, that the design and construction meet applicable standards, that its operators are fully trained to carry out their tasks, and that operating plans and procedures give all necessary attention to the requirements of radiation safety. The terms and conditions of licensing are likely to change as new information and experience become available. Licensed facilities should be obliged to comply with such changes as a condition of continued approval.

Operating controls

A plant that has been licensed to irradiate food should be subject to regular quality control and quality assurance procedures to verify that the plant is operating according to the licence agreement. These performance checks should examine the quality of the products being irradiated, ensure that the proper dose of radiation is being delivered for the intended effect, and verify that irradiation procedures are being followed scrupulously. The irradiation process must incorporate appropriate safety arrangements. The source (isotope or electron beam) must be placed within a biological shield — a building of concrete which completely surrounds the irradiation unit with walls of such thickness that there is no possibility of radiation exposure outside the shield. The isotope radiation source, when not in use, should be stored in a deep tank of water or a dry storage container which absorbs the radiation. A series of fail-safe procedures is needed to ensure that the isotope cannot be raised into the working position or the electron beam switched on if any person is in a position to be exposed to any radiation.

The trained technical staff of an irradiation plant who have to enter the irradiation room for maintenance or repair, and who theoretically could be exposed to radiation, should carry dosimeters with them. Regular evaluation of the dosimeter records and medical surveillance will ensure that these workers never receive an exposure above the maximum permissible level. Internationally recognized guidelines for radiation protection have been established by the International Committee for Radiological Protection.

In addition to internal monitoring, each food irradiation plant should be subject to both regularly scheduled and unannounced inspections by government personnel to make sure that they comply with the terms of their licences and with applicable regulations. Government regulatory agencies can often provide technical guidance and training to help these plants maintain high standards and apply new technical and scientific information.

Criteria and standards

The Codex General Standard for Irradiated Foods (see Annex 2) and the Recommended International Code of Practice for the Operation of Irradiation Facilities Used for the Treatment of Food (see Annex 3) provide authoritative guidelines that are recognized by regulatory authorities and industry around the world as a basis for safe and effective radiation practices. Irradiation facilities that process food are also covered by the General Principles of Food Hygiene, prepared by the FAO/WHO Codex Alimentarius Commission as a basic recommendation to ensure hygienic food handling and processing. In addition, all the Codex Codes of hygiene and/or technological practice elaborated for specific food commodities will apply as appropriate. Together with legislation and regulations adopted by countries that have approved the use of radiation in the processing of food, these recognized standards will help to ensure that the benefits of this technique will be safely and productively realized by people throughout the world.

National regulatory bodies throughout the world, United Nations agencies, and the food industry are taking an approach based on scientific information, extensive experience, and a genuine regard for the needs and concerns of the general public.

Chapter 6

CONSUMER ACCEPTANCE

One of the main reasons why food irradiation is not yet in more general use is that governments are uncertain of consumer acceptance of irradiated foods. Without public endorsement, food irradiation will remain largely neglected not only in the developed world but also in developing countries, which are reluctant to invest in expensive plant and equipment when developed countries seem to be unenthusiastic. Although some 34 countries have granted approval for radiation processing of about 30 food products, industry has been slow to expand the use of radiation. This is true despite the safety and effectiveness of the process, and despite evidence that irradiation is cost-effective in controlling harmful organisms and extending shelf-life.

The failure of food irradiation to gain wider acceptance is not difficult to fathom. Negative public attitudes towards virtually everything associated with radiation are found all over the world. In millions of people's minds radiation is associated with war on a scale the earth has never seen, with accidents that pose health threats lasting for generations, and with nuclear wastes that will still be dangerous 10 000 years from now. Even recognizing that radiation is an invaluable aid in diagnosing and treating disease, sterilizing medical devices and pharmaceutical products, and producing many kinds of manufactured goods, vast numbers of people are genuinely afraid of anything that would appear to increase the risk of exposure to radiation.

In addition, there is apparently wide public misunderstanding of what the process is, how it works, and what it will and will not do. A major misconception is that food processed by radiation becomes radioactive. But there are other concerns based on misunderstanding or lack of information that needlessly stand in the way of effective use of this procedure.

What follows is a series of questions and answers that address the most common concerns, fears and misapprehensions about food irradiation. They are couched in non-technical terms in order to be readily understandable to consumers (the bibliography lists many references to further reading for those interested in more detailed information on food irradiation).

Following the questions and answers is a brief discussion of the approaches that governments, industry, consumer organizations, the media, the health and education communities, and others might well consider in order to achieve broader public acceptance of food irradiation.

* * * * *

What is done to food when it is irradiated?

The food is exposed to a form of energy called ionizing radiation, the same kind of energy used to make X-ray pictures, sterilize up to 50% of all disposable medical and hygienic products, treat certain kinds of cancer, and for many other purposes.

Why is food treated with radiation?

Food is irradiated for the same reasons that it is processed by heat or refrigeration or freezing or treated with chemicals — to kill insects, fungi, and bacteria that cause food to spoil and can cause disease, and to make it possible to keep it longer and in better condition in warehouses, stores, and homes.

Is irradiated food safe to eat?

Yes. The treatment does not alter the food in any way that could harm people.

Does irradiation make food radioactive?

No, food irradiated under approved conditions does not become radioactive.

But do irradiated foods look or smell or taste different?

Because of the small amount of energy involved in food irradiation, usually no significant difference in terms of appearance, smell, or taste can be detected if the process has been carried out properly. It is even difficult to detect any change by means of analysis in a laboratory. It is worth remembering that food processors want their products to appeal to consumers, not put them off. If an irradiated food product were very different from what consumers expect, there would be no market for it.

Are irradiated foods still nutritious?

Yes. Irradiation, like all known methods of processing food, can lower the content of some nutrients, such as vitamins, but storing food at room temperature for a few hours after harvesting does the same thing. At low doses of radiation, nutrient losses are either not measurable or, if they can be measured, are not significant. At the higher doses used to extend shelf-life or control harmful bacteria, nutritional losses are less than, or about the same as, those caused by other kinds of food processing. It can certainly be said that irradiated foods are wholesome and nutritious.

Are there long-term effects of eating irradiated foods?

Studies in animals, many of which continued for periods of years, have not disclosed any reason to be concerned about long-term health effects of irradiated food or about risks from eating such food. These studies have been conducted in many different countries and by reputable international organizations.

But didn't some animal tests fail to show that food irradiation is safe?

Over the last 30 years, many hundreds of tests have been carried out with animals fed irradiated foods or components of irradiated foods. A very small number of these tests gave inconclusive results that were interpreted as showing that food irradiation is unsafe. Each of these studies has been thoroughly reviewed and, in many cases, repeated. The results of these follow-up investigations provided explanations for the original "negative" findings. Usually the problem lay in the design of the study or the way it was conducted. Sometimes the sample size — the number of animals used in the study — was too small to allow the results to be interpreted properly. In other instances, the repeat studies were simply unable to reproduce the original results. In fact, more than 100 generations of sensitive laboratory animals in the United Kingdom alone have been living and prospering on diets sterilized by irradiation. Similar results have been obtained in many other countries.

What are "radiolytic products"?

This is a scientific term meaning chemical compounds formed by exposure to ionizing radiation. Such compounds are formed in food processed by radiation and they are identical or similar to compounds found in food processed by other techniques, such as cooking, or even in unprocessed foods.

Have all radiolytic products in food been identified, and are any of them dangerous?

Extensive research has been done to identify and evaluate radiolytic products in food. No one can say with certainty that all such products have been found, but the important finding is that all those identified so far are similar to compounds commonly found in food. They are not unique in the sense that they occur only as a result of irradiation. And, moreover, there is no evidence that any of these substances poses a danger to human health.

Could some of them be damaging cells without our knowing it?

Again, the answer is no. Chemicals and other agents capable of damaging cells are called mutagens. Our food, irradiated or not, naturally contains some mutagens. They can be formed by conventional food processing methods whose safety is accepted. Smoked foods, for example, may contain chemicals that can injure cells. But, despite extensive studies, there is no evidence that irradiated foods present any increased risk of exposure to mutagens than do conventionally processed foods.

What about the microorganisms in food that irradiation doesn't kill. Are they more dangerous?

It is true that irradiation — at the levels normally used in food processing — does not destroy every single microorganism present; it does not sterilize the food. After treatment, the surviving organisms may start to multiply again if conditions are favourable. For example, the spores of the bacterium known as *Clostridium botulinum* are not killed by low doses of radiation. If irradiated or heat-pasteurized food containing this organism is kept in a sealed container at room temperature, *C. botulinum* can multiply and produce the toxin that causes botulism, a frequently fatal form of foodborne disease. It is important to remember that surviving pathogens in irradiated food are just as dangerous — but no more so — as the same organisms in unirradiated food. As with any food, consumers must take appropriate precautions, such as refrigeration and proper handling and cooking, to make sure that potentially harmful organisms do not present a problem.

What foods are treated with radiation?

Certainly not all foods, and in fact not even most of them, are now or will be candidates for treatment with radiation. The technique is used only when needed and only when it is economically advantageous. Some examples of foods that have been approved for radiation treatment in a number of countries are listed below:

- potatoes and onions — to control sprouting when climatic conditions make storage difficult;
- spices, herbs, dehydrated vegetables, and condiments — to control microorganisms and get rid of insects;

Food irradiation

> poultry, shrimps, frog legs, and fish — to control microorganisms (in particular pathogens) and prolong shelf-life;
>
> mangoes, papayas, strawberries, and mushrooms — to control insects and to extend shelf-life;
>
> rice, cocoa beans and wheat — to control insects and microorganisms.

The fact that approval has been granted for radiation processing of certain foods does not necessarily mean that the local product will be irradiated. The choice depends on many factors, such as availability of alternative processing methods and especially cost. But if the product is destined for export, it is more likely that irradiation treatment will be used because of its effectiveness in controlling insect pests and extending shelf-life. If the particular product gives rise to a public health problem (e.g., raw poultry), radiation treatment is quite likely to be used because, in contrast to other methods of processing such as heat, it leaves the product unchanged.

Are irradiated foods on the market now?

Irradiation of food has been approved in 33 countries for some 30 food products (see Annex 1), and the list is increasing all the time. In some countries, approval is only for testing purposes, to work out the appropriate dose for a given kind of food. Test marketing has been carried out in some countries, and a few countries have had irradiated food products on the market for a number of years, but there is not yet a big commercial market for irradiated food.

One reason for this, especially as far as local and national marketing is concerned, is the lack of consumer understanding and acceptance of food irradiation. This barrier is gradually being lowered as governments, consumer organizations, and others provide information that helps consumers make informed judgements about the value of food irradiation, and organize test marketing trials to enable consumers to evaluate the quality and benefits of irradiated foods.

Who regulates and inspects food irradiation facilities?

Enforcement of health and safety standards will, of course, vary from country to country. A facility would need to register as a food-processing establishment and to obtain a licence from the government body concerned with regulating and inspecting the food industry to ensure that basic hygienic requirements are being met. Approval to handle radioactive materials usually comes from a country's atomic energy authority. Once licensed and in operation the irradiation unit would probably have to operate in accordance with the guidelines recommended by the Codex Alimentarius

Commission (see Annexes 2 and 3). Enforcement of those guidelines would be the responsibility of the government body concerned with regulating and inspecting the food processing industry. There may never be an international monitoring programme, but the International Atomic Energy Agency plans to publish a list of accredited food irradiation establishments and FAO will continue to include information on food irradiation in its technical manuals.

How can irradiated foods be identified in the market?

Irradiated foods cannot be recognized by sight, smell, taste, or feel. The only sure way for consumers to know if a food has been processed by irradiation is for the product to carry a label that clearly announces the treatment in words, a symbol, or both. Labelling practices can be expected to vary from country to country, but countries that elect to follow the guidelines developed by the Codex Alimentarius Commission[1] will label all foods that have been irradiated and, in addition, possibly other products that have not themselves been irradiated, but of which one or more components were irradiated before incorporation into the final product. The choice of wording, or symbol, is up to the individual country. However, the symbol shown in Fig. 4 is gaining increasing acceptance as a means of informing the public that a food product has been treated with ionizing radiation.

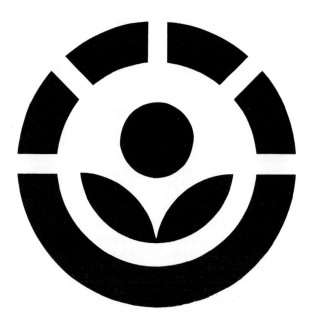

Fig. 4. Symbol indicating that a food product has been treated with ionizing radiation.

Food irradiation

The need for labelling and public information

It has been suggested that irrradiated food should not be specially labelled, the argument being that other forms of food processing are not identified on the label, that irradiated food does not present any hazard that people need to be aware of, and that consumers might hesitate to buy food products identified with the word "irradiated", especially since in some languages there is little distinction between "irradiated" and "contaminated" (with radioactive pollutants). They also argue that the word "irradiated" by itself does not give sufficient information on the benefits of food irradiation.

Proposals not to label irradiated food have generally been rejected in favour of providing full information, on the grounds that consumers have a right to be informed about the food products they buy and use. The facts that the technique is safe and effective and that irradiated foods are wholesome and pose no threat to health are not grounds for secrecy. A policy of non-disclosure would in the long run discourage the use of radiation processing, rather than encourage it. Informed consumers might in future give preference to irradiated poultry, to give just one example, in order to be sure of buying food free from pathogens.

To be of genuine value to consumers, labelling of irradiated food must be supported by public information and education campaigns designed initially to help consumers decide whether they want to be able to buy radiation-processed foods and subsequently to help them make wise decisions in the selection and use of irradiated food products. Countries will, of course, mount public education efforts according to their individual needs, resources, and policies. In some circumstances, the government will be the main, perhaps the sole, source of information. In others, the food industry, consumer groups, and the media will be active in public information and education programmes, and, hopefully, all will collaborate to provide reliable and useful information to the public. National steering committees composed of representatives of all interests could prove most useful in coordinating educational activities, by ensuring that the information materials developed and distributed to the public are accurate, comprehensive, and consistent.

The individuals and bodies who are already convinced that food irradiation can make a great contribution towards reducing food losses and preventing foodborne disease are understandably eager to see a rapid expansion of radiation food processing. These benefits seem, in the minds of many, to represent a powerful argument in favour of food irradiation. But it is vital to remember that consumers are no longer willing to accept such arguments passively, and will insist upon being fully involved in any decision made about food irradiation. They will certainly request full and factual information about the scientific rationale for using ionizing radiation, as well as an obligation to provide clear labelling of irradiated food products.

Countries that contemplate launching or expanding the use of radiation food processing should be prepared to seek full consumer participation in pursuing this course of action. Effective public information and education are essential steps in that process.

BIBLIOGRAPHY

General

BROWNWELL, L.E. *Radiation uses in industry and science.* Washington, DC, US Atomic Energy Commission, US Government Printing Office, 1961.

ELIAS, P.S. & COHEN, A.J., ed. *Recent advances in food irradiation.* Amsterdam, Elsevier, 1983.

Food irradiation. Japan, Japanese Research Association for Food Irradiation, 1982.

Food irradiation now. Proceedings of a Symposium, The Hague, Martinus Nijhoff/Dr W. Junk Publishers, 1982.

HANNAN, R.S. *Scientific and technological problems involved in using ionizing radiation for the preservation of food.* London, Her Majesty's Stationery Office, 1955 (Department of Scientific and Industrial Research Food Investigation, Special Report No. 61).

JOSEPHSON, E.S. & PETERSON, M.S., ed. *Preservation of food by ionizing radiation,* Vol. I, II, III. Boca Raton, Florida, CRC Press, 1982, 1983.

Radiation preservation of food. Washington, DC, US Army Quartermaster Corps, US Government Printing Office, 1957.

URBAIN, W.M. *Food irradiation.* New York, Academic Press, 1986.

The process of food irradiation

BECKER, R.L. Absence of induced radioactivity in irradiated foods. In: Elias, P.S. & Cohen, A.J., ed., *Recent advances in food irradiation.* Amsterdam, Elsevier Biomedical, 1983.

BROWNELL, L.E. *Radiation uses in industry and science.* Washington, DC, US Government Printing Office, 1961.

BRYNJOLFSSON, A. & WANG, C.P. Atomic structure. In: Josephson, E.S. & Peterson, M.S., ed. *Preservation of food by ionizing radiation,* Vol. I. Boca Raton, Florida, CRC Press, 1983.

CHARLESBY, A., ed. *Radiation sources.* New York, Macmillan, 1964.

HURST, G.S. & TURNER, J.E. *Elementary radiation physics.* New York, Wiley, 1970.

IAEA. *Dosimetry in agriculture, industry, biology and medicine.* Vienna, International Atomic Energy Agency, 1973.

IAEA. *Manual of food irradiation dosimetry.* Vienna, International Atomic Energy Agency, 1977 (Technical Report Series No. 178).

IAEA. *Training manual on food irradiation technology and techniques,* 2nd ed. Vienna, International Atomic Energy Agency, 1982 (Technical Report Series No. 114).

Radionuclides in foods. Washington, DC, National Academy of Sciences, 1973.

WANG, C.P. & BRYNJOLFSSON, A. Interactions of charged particles and γ-rays with matter. In: Josephson, E.S. & Peterson, M.S., ed. *Preservation of food by ionizing radiation,* Vol. I. Boca Raton, Florida, CRC Press, 1983.

WANG, Y., ed. *Handbook of radioactive nuclides.* Boca Raton, Florida, CRC Press, 1969.

Effects of food irradiation

BASSON, R.A. Chemiclearance, *Nuclear active (South Africa),* **17**: 3 (1977).

CHAUHAN, P. *Assessment of irradiated foods for toxicological safety - newer methods.* Karlsruhe, International Project in the Field of Food Irradiation (IPFFI), 1974 (Food Irradiation Information No. 3).

CODEX ALIMENTARIUS COMMISSION. *The microbiological safety of irradiated food.* Report of a Meeting of the Board of the International Committee on Food Microbiology and Hygiene of the International Union of Microbiological Societies with the participation of WHO, FAO, and IAEA. Rome, Codex Alimentarius Commission, FAO, 1982.

ELIAS, P.S. & COHEN, A.J. *Radiation chemistry of major food components.* Amsterdam, Elsevier Biomedical, 1977.

Fourth activity report. Karlsruhe, International Project in the Field of Food Irradiation (IPFFI), 1981.

Ionizing energy in food processing and pest control. 1. Wholesomeness of food treated with ionizing energy. Ames, Iowa, Council for Agricultural Science and Technology (CAST), 1986.

Is radiation food additive?. Ames, Iowa, Council for Agricultural Science and Technology (CAST), 1984.

JOSEPHSON, E.S. ET AL. Nutritional aspects of food irradiation: an overview. *Journal of food processing and preservation,* **2**: 299 (1978).

Recommendations for evaluating the safety of irradiated foods. Washington, DC, Report of the Irradiated Foods Committee, US Food and Drug Administration, 1980.

WHO Technical Report Series, No. 659, 1980 *(Wholesomeness of irradiated food:* report of a Joint FAO/IAEA/WHO Expert Committee).

Practical applications of food irradiation

CHARLESBY, A. *Radiation sources.* Oxford, Pergamon, 1964.

DOLLSTÄDT, R. A new onion irradiator, *Food irradiation newsletter,* **8**: 40 (1984).

Food irradiation prospects for Canadian technology development: a statement. Ottawa, Science Council of Canada, 1987.

FRAZER, F.M. Gamma radiation processing equipment and associated energy requirements in food irradiation. In: *Combination process in food irradiation.* Vienna, International Atomic Energy Agency, 1981.

GAY, R.G. Design and operation of radiation facilities. In: *Ionizing energy treatment of foods, Proceedings of a Symposium.* Sydney, 1983.

Handbook for conducting feasibility studies. Vienna, International Consultative Group on Food Irradiation, International Atomic Energy Agency, 1986.

Legislation in the field of food irradiation. Vienna, International Atomic Energy Agency, 1987 (IAEA-TECDOC-422).

MILLS, S. *Issues in food irradiation: a discussion paper.* Ottawa, Science Council of Canada, 1987.

MORRISON, R.M. & ROBERTS, T. *Food irradiation: new perspectives on a controversial technology.* Washington, DC, Congress of the United States, Office of Technology Assessment, 1985.

Radiation pasteurizing fresh strawberries and other fresh fruits and vegetables: estimates of costs and benefits. Washington, DC, US Atomic Energy Commission, 1965.

The commercial prospects of selected irradiated foods. Washington, DC, US Department of Commerce, 1968 (TID 24058).

Trade promotion of irradiated food. Vienna, International Atomic Energy Agency, 1986 (IAEA-TECDOC-391).

UMEDA, K. Commercial experience with the Shihoro Potato Irradiator. *Food irradiation newsletter,* **7**(2): 19 (1983).

URBAIN, W.M. Review of factors and conditions influencing the economics of food irradiation applications. *Food irradiation newsletter,* **7**(1): 36 (1983).

VAN DER LINDE, H.J. Economic considerations for the irradiation preservation of foods in South Africa. *Food irradiation newsletter,* **7**(3): 32 (1983).

WHO. *Task Force meeting on the use of irradiation to ensure hygienic quality of food.* World Health Organization, Geneva, 1987 (unpublished document WHO/EHE/FOS/87.2).

Legislation and control of food irradiation

Codex general standard for the labelling of prepackaged foods. Rome, Codex Alimentarius Commission, FAO, 1987 (CAC/Vol. VI-Ed. 2).

Food irradiation: some regulatory and technical aspects. Vienna, International Atomic Energy Agency, 1985 (IAEA-TECDOC-349).

International acceptance of irradiated food. Legal aspect. Vienna, International Atomic Energy Agency, 1979.

Irradiated foods for human consumption. *Federal register,* **46** (59): 18992-18994 (1981).

LADOMERY, L.G. & NOCERA, F. Technical and legal aspects relating to labelling of irradiated food stuffs. *Food irradiation newsletter,* **4**: 32 (1980).

Legislation in the field of food irradiation. Vienna, International Atomic Energy Agency, 1987 (IAEA-TECDOC-422).

Recommended international code of practice: general principles of food hygiene. Rome, Codex Alimentarius Commission, FAO, 1983 (CAC/Vol. A-Ed. 1).

WHO Technical Report Series, No. 604, 1977. (*Wholesomeness of irradiated food:* report of a Joint FAO/IAEA/WHO Expert Committee).

WHO Technical Report Series, No. 659, 1981. (*Wholesomeness of irradiated food:* report of a Joint FAO/IAEA/WHO Expert Committee).

Consumer acceptance

Consumer reaction to the irradiation concept. Albuquerque, New Mexico, US Department of Energy and National Pork Producers Council, 1984.

DEFESCHE, F. How does the consumer react to irradiated food? In: *Food irradiation now.* The Hague, Martinus Nijhoff/Dr W. Junk, 1982.

IAEA. *Marketing and consumer acceptance of irradiated foods.* Report of Consultants' Meeting. Vienna, International Atomic Energy Agency, 1983 (IAEA-TECDOC-290).

Marketability testing of irradiated fish and seafood. Concept development and testing. Ottawa, Department of Fisheries and Oceans, 1984.

URBAIN, R.W. & URBAIN, W.M. Marketing and labelling of radiation insect-disinfested foods. In: Moy, J.H., ed. *Radiation disinfestation of food and agricultural products.* Honolulu, University of Hawaii Press, 1985.

URBAIN W.M. Radiation update. In: *Feeding the military man.* Natick, Massachusetts, US Army Natick Laboratories, 1970.

VAN DER LINDE, H.J. Marketing experience with radurized products in South Africa. In: *Ionizing energy treatment of food. Proceedings of a Symposium.* Sydney, 1983.

VAN KOOIJ, J.G. Consumer attitudes toward food irradiation in the Netherlands. In: *Requirements for the irradiation of food on a commercial scale.* Vienna, International Atomic Energy Agency, 1975.

Publications and documents prepared by the International Atomic Energy Agency, Vienna.

Application of food irradiation in developing countries (1966).

Aspects of the introduction of food irradiation in developing countries (1973).

Combination processes in food irradiation (1981).

Decontamination of animal feeds by irradiation (1979).

Disinfestation of fruit by irradiation (1971).

Elimination of harmful organisms from food and feed by irradiation (1968).

Enzymological aspects of food irradiation (1969).

Factors influencing the economical application of food irradiation (1973).

Improvement of food quality by irradiation (1974).

Microbiological problems in food preservation by irradiation (1967).

Microbiological specifications and testing methods for irradiated food (1970).

Preservation of fish by irradiation (1970).

Preservation of fruit and vegetables by radiation (1968).

Radiation control of salmonellae in food and feed products (1963).

Radurization of scampi, shrimp and cod (1971).

Requirement for the irradiation of food on a commercial scale (1975).

Training manual on food irradiation technology and techniques (2nd ed., 1982).

In addition, the IAEA publishes proceedings of symposia and seminars on food irradiation, among them the following:

Food irradiation, Proceedings of a Symposium, Karlsruhe, 1966.

Radiation preservation of food, Proceedings of a Symposium, Bombay, 1973.

Food preservation by irradiation, Vols. I and II. Proceedings of a Symposium, Wageningen, 1977.

International Symposium on Food Irradiation Processing, Washington, DC, 1985.

Food irradiation for developing countries in Asia and the Pacific, Proceedings of a seminar, IAEA-TECDOC-271, Tokyo, 1981.

Marketing and consumer acceptance of irradiated foods, Report of a Consultants' Meeting, IAEA-TECDOC-290, Vienna, 1982.

Use of irradiation as a quarantine treatment of agricultural commodities, IAEA-TECDOC-326, Honolulu, 1983.

Annex 1

LIST OF COUNTRIES THAT HAVE CLEARED IRRADIATED FOOD FOR HUMAN CONSUMPTION

(Updated 22 March 1988)

Country	Product	Purpose of irradiation	Type of clearance	Dose permitted (kGy)	Date of approval
Argentina	strawberries	shelf-life extension	unconditional	2.5 max.	30 April 1987
	potatoes	sprout inhibition	unconditional	0.03 to 0.15	30 April 1987
	onions	sprout inhibition	unconditional	0.02 to 0.15	30 April 1987
	garlic	sprout inhibition	unconditional	0.02 to 0.15	30 April 1987
Bangladesh	chicken	shelf-life extension/decontamination	unconditional	up to 8	28 December 1983
	papaya	insect disinfestation/control of ripening	unconditional	up to 1	28 December 1983
	potatoes	sprout inhibition	unconditional	up to 0.15	28 December 1983
	wheat and ground wheat products	insect disinfestation	unconditional	up to 1	28 December 1983
	fish	shelf-life extension/decontamination/insect disinfestation	unconditional	up to 2.2	28 December 1983
	onions	sprout inhibition	unconditional	up to 0.15	28 December 1983
	rice	insect disinfestation	unconditional	up to 1	28 December 1983
	frog legs	decontamination	provisional		
	shrimp	shelf-life extension/decontamination	provisional		
	mangoes	shelf-life extension/insect disinfestation/control ripening	unconditional	up to 1	28 December 1983
	pulses	insect disinfestation	unconditional	up to 1	28 December 1983
	spices	decontamination/insect disinfestation	unconditional	up to 10	28 December 1983
Belgium	potatoes	sprout inhibition	provisional	up to 0.15	16 July 1980
	strawberries	shelf-life extension	provisional	up to 3	16 July 1980
	onions	sprout inhibition	provisional	up to 0.15	16 October 1980
	garlic	sprout inhibition	provisional	up to 0.15	16 October 1980
	shallots	sprout inhibition	provisional	up to 0.15	16 October 1980
	black/white pepper	decontamination	provisional	up to 10	16 October 1980
	paprika powder	decontamination	provisional	up to 10	16 October 1980
	arabic gum	decontamination	provisional	up to 10	29 September 1983
	spices (78 different products)	decontamination	provisional	up to 10	29 September 1983
	(semi)-dried vegetables (7 different products)	decontamination	provisional	up to 10	29 September 1983

Annex 1

Country	Product	Purpose of irradiation	Type of clearance	Dose permitted (kGy)	Date of approval
Brazil	rice	insect disinfestation	unconditional	up to 1	7 March 1985
	potatoes	sprout inhibition	unconditional	up to 0.15	7 March 1985
	onions	sprout inhibition	unconditional	up to 0.15	7 March 1985
	beans	insect disinfestation	unconditional	up to 1	7 March 1985
	maize	insect disinfestation	unconditional	up to 0.5	7 March 1985
	wheat	insect disinfestation	unconditional	up to 1	7 March 1985
	wheat flour	insect disinfestation	unconditional	up to 1	7 March 1985
	spices (13 different products)	decontamination/insect disinfestation	unconditional	up to 10	7 March 1985
	papaya	insect disinfestation/control of ripening	unconditional	up to 1	7 March 1985
	strawberries	shelf-life extension	unconditional	up to 3	7 March 1985
	fish and fish products (fillets, salted, smoked dried, dehydrated)	shelf-life extension/decontamination/insect disinfestation	unconditional	up to 2.2	8 March 1985
	poultry	shelf-life extension/decontamination	unconditional	up to 7	8 March 1985
Bulgaria	potatoes	sprout inhibition	experimental batches	0.1	30 April 1972
	onions	sprout inhibition	experimental batches	0.1	30 April 1972
	garlic	sprout inhibition	experimental batches	0.1	30 April 1972
	grain	insect disinfestation	experimental batches	0.3	30 April 1972
	dry food concentrates	insect disinfestation	experimental batches	1	30 April 1972
	dried fruits	insect disinfestation	experimental batches	1	30 April 1972
	fresh fruits (tomatoes, peaches, apricots, cherries, raspberries, grapes)	shelf-life extension	experimental batches	2.5	30 April 1972
Canada	potatoes	sprout inhibition	unconditional	up to 0.1	9 November 1960
	onions	sprout inhibition	unconditional	up to 0.15	14 June 1963
	wheat, flour, wholewheat	insect disinfestation	unconditional	up to 0.75	25 March 1965
	poultry	decontamination	test marketing	up to 7	25 February 1969
	cod and haddock fillets	shelf-life extension	test marketing	up to 1.5	20 June 1973
					2 October 1973
	spices and certain dried vegetables' seasonings	decontamination	unconditional	up to 10	3 October 1984
	onion powder	decontamination	unconditional	up to 10	12 December 1983

63

Food irradiation

Country	Product	Purpose of irradiation	Type of clearance	Dose permitted (kGy)	Date of approval
Chile	potatoes	sprout inhibition	experimental batches test marketing		31 October 1974
			unconditional	up to 0.15	29 December 1982
	papaya	insect disinfestation	unconditional	up to 1	29 December 1982
	wheat and ground wheat products	insect disinfestation	unconditional	up to 1	29 December 1982
	strawberries	shelf-life extension	unconditional	up to 3	29 December 1982
	chicken	decontamination	unconditional	up to 7	29 December 1982
	onions	sprout inhibition	unconditional	up to 0.15	29 December 1982
	rice	insect disinfestation	unconditional	up to 1	29 December 1982
	teleost fish and fish products	shelf-life extension/decontamination/insect disinfestation	unconditional	up to 2.2	29 December 1982
	cocoa beans	decontamination/insect disinfestation	unconditional	up to 5	29 December 1982
	dates	insect disinfestation	unconditional	up to 1	29 December 1982
	mangoes	shelf-life extension/insect disinfestation/control of ripening	unconditional	up to 1	29 December 1982
	pulses	insect disinfestation	unconditional	up to 1	29 December 1982
	spices and condiments	decontamination/insect disinfestation	unconditional	up to 10	29 December 1982
China	potatoes	sprout inhibition	unconditional	up to 0.20	30 November 1984
	onions	sprout inhibition	unconditional	up to 0.15	30 November 1984
	garlic	sprout inhibition	unconditional	up to 0.10	30 November 1984
	peanuts	insect disinfestation	unconditional	up to 0.40	30 November 1984
	grain	insect disinfestation	unconditional	up to 0.45	30 November 1984
	mushrooms	growth inhibition	unconditional	up to 1	30 November 1984
	sausage	decontamination	unconditional	up to 8	30 November 1984
Czechoslovakia	potatoes	sprout inhibition	experimental batches	up to 0.1	26 November 1976
	onions	sprout inhibition	experimental batches	up to 0.08	26 November 1976
	mushrooms	growth inhibition	experimental	up to 2	26 November 1976
Denmark	spices and herbs	decontamination	unconditional	up to 15 max. up to 10 average	23 December 1985
Finland	dry and dehydrated spices and herbs	decontamination	unconditional	up to 10 average	13 November 1987
	all foods for patients requiring a sterile diet	sterilization	unconditional	unlimited	13 November 1987
France	potatoes	sprout inhibition	provisional	0.075—0.15	8 November 1972
	onions	sprout inhibition	provisional	0.075—0.15	9 August 1977
	garlic	sprout inhibition	provisional	0.075—0.15	9 August 1977

Annex 1

Country	Product	Purpose of irradiation	Type of clearance	Dose permitted (kGy)	Date of approval
	shallots	sprout inhibition	provisional	0.075–0.15	9 August 1977
	spices and aromatic substances (72 products including powdered onion and garlic)	decontamination	unconditional	up to 11	10 February 1983
	gum arabic	decontamination	unconditional	up to 9	16 June 1985
	muesli-like cereal	decontamination	unconditional	up to 10	16 June 1985
	dehydrated vegetables	decontamination	unconditional	up to 10	16 June 1985
	mechanically deboned poultry meat	decontamination	unconditional	up to 5	16 February 1985
	dried fruits	insect disinfestation	unconditional	1 max.	6 January 1988
	dried vegetables	insect disinfestation	unconditional	1 max.	6 January 1988
German Democratic Republic	onions	sprout inhibition	test marketing	50	1981
	onions	sprout inhibition	unconditional	20	30 January 1984
	enzyme solutions	decontamination	unconditional	10	7 June 1983
	spices	decontamination	provisional	up to 10	29 December 1982
Hungary	potatoes	sprout inhibition	test marketing	0.1	23 December 1969
	potatoes	sprout inhibition	test marketing	0.15 max.	10 January 1972
	potatoes	sprout inhibition	test marketing	0.15 max.	5 March 1973
	onions	sprout inhibition	test marketing		5 March 1973
	strawberries	shelf-life extension	test marketing		5 March 1973
	mixed spices (black pepper, cumin, paprika, dried garlic: for use in sausages)	decontamination	experimental batches	5	2 April 1974
	onions	sprout inhibition	test marketing	0.06	6 August 1975
	onions	sprout inhibition	experimental batches	0.06	6 September 1976
	mixed dry ingredients for canned hashed meat	decontamination	experimental batches	5	20 November 1976
	potatoes	sprout inhibition	test marketing	0.10	4 May 1980
	onions (for dehydrated flakes processing)	sprout inhibition	experimental batches	0.05	15 September 1980
	mushrooms (*Agaricus*)	growth inhibition	test marketing	0.05	18 November 1980
	strawberries	shelf-life extension	test marketing	2.5	20 June 1981
	potatoes	sprout inhibition	test marketing	2.5	20 June 1981
	potatoes	sprout inhibition	test marketing	0.1	13 October 1981
	spices for sausage production	decontamination	test marketing	0.10	2 December 1981
	strawberries	shelf-life extension	test marketing	5	4 January 1982
	mushrooms (*Agaricus*)	growth inhibition	test marketing	2.5	15 April 1982
	mushrooms (*Pleurotus*)	growth inhibition	test marketing	3	15 April 1982

Food irradiation

Country	Product	Purpose of irradiation	Type of clearance	Dose permitted (kGy)	Date of approval
Hungary (contd)	grapes	shelf-life extension	test marketing	2.5	15 April 1982
	cherries	shelf-life extension	test marketing	2.5	15 April 1982
	sour cherries	shelf-life extension	test marketing	2.5	15 April 1982
	red currants	shelf-life extension	test marketing	2.5	15 April 1982
	onions	sprout inhibition	unconditional	0.05 ± 0.02	23 June 1982
	spices for sausage	decontamination	test marketing	5	28 June 1982
	pears	shelf-life extension	test marketing	2.5	7 December 1982
	pears	shelf-life extension	test marketing	1.0 + $CaCl_2$ treatment	24 January 1983
	spices	decontamination	test marketing	5	1983
	potatoes (for processing into flakes)	sprout inhibition	test marketing	0.1	28 January 1983
	frozen chicken	decontamination	test marketing	4	3 October 1983
	sour cherries (canned)		conditional	0.2 average	20 February 1984
	black pepper	decontamination	conditional	6 minimum	23 April 1985
	spices	decontamination	conditional	5–6 minimum	May 1985
	spices	decontamination	unconditional	8, 6 average	25 April 1986
India	potatoes	sprout inhibition	unconditional	Codex Standard	January 1986
	onions	sprout inhibition	unconditional	Codex Standard	January 1986
	spices	disinfection	for export only	Codex Standard	January 1986
	frozen shrimps and frog legs	disinfection	for export only	Codex Standard	January 1986
Indonesia	dried spices	decontamination	unconditional	10 max.	29 December 1987
	tuber and root crops (potatoes, shallots, garlic and rhizomes)	sprout inhibition	unconditional	0.15 max.	29 December 1987
	cereals	disinfestation	unconditional	1 max.	29 December 1987
Israel	potatoes	sprout inhibition	unconditional	0.15 max.	5 July 1967
	onions	sprout inhibition	unconditional	0.10 max.	25 July 1968
	poultry and poultry sections	shelf-life extension/decontamination	unconditional	7 max.	23 April 1982
	onions	sprout inhibition	unconditional	0.15	6 March 1985
	garlic	sprout inhibition	unconditional	0.15	6 March 1985
	shallots	sprout inhibition	unconditional	0.15	6 March 1985
	spices (36 different products)	decontamination	unconditional	10	6 March 1985
	fresh fruits and vegetables	disinfestation	unconditional	1 average	January 1987
	grains, cereals, pulses, cocoa & coffee beans, nuts, edible seeds	disinfestation	unconditional	1 average	January 1987

Annex 1

Country	Product	Purpose of irradiation	Type of clearance	Dose permitted (kGy)	Date of approval
	mushrooms, strawberries	shelf-life extension	unconditional	3 average	January 1987
	poultry and poultry sections	decontamination	unconditional	7 average	January 1987
	spices & condiments, dehydrated & dried vegetables, edible herbs	decontamination	unconditional	10 average	January 1987
	poultry feeds	decontamination	unconditional	15 average	January 1987
Italy	potatoes	sprout inhibition	unconditional	0.075−0.15	30 August 1973
	onions	sprout inhibition	unconditional	0.075−0.15	30 August 1973
	garlic	sprout inhibition	unconditional	0.075−0.15	30 August 1973
Japan	potatoes	sprout inhibition	unconditional	0.15 max.	30 August 1972
Netherlands	asparagus	shelf-life extension/growth inhibition	experimental batches	2 max.	7 May 1969
	cocoa beans	insect disinfestation	experimental batches	0.7 max.	7 May 1969
	strawberries	shelf-life extension	experimental batches	2.5 max.	7 May 1969
	mushrooms	growth inhibition	unconditional	2.5 max.	23 October 1969
	deep frozen meals	sterilization	hospital patients	25 min.	27 November 1969
	potatoes	sprout inhibition	unconditional	0.15 max.	23 March 1970
	shrimps	shelf-life extension	experimental batches	0.5−1	13 November 1970
	onions	sprout inhibition	experimental batches	0.15	5 February 1971
	spices and condiments	decontamination	experimental batches	8−10	13 September 1971
	poultry, eviscerated (in plastic bags)	shelf-life extension	experimental batches	3 max.	31 December 1971
	chicken	shelf-life extension/decontamination	unconditional	3 max.	10 May 1976
	fresh, tinned and liquid foodstuffs	sterilization	hospital patients	25 min.	8 March 1972
	spices	decontamination	provisional	10	4 October 1974
	powdered batter mix	decontamination	test marketing	1.5	4 October 1974
	vegetable filling	decontamination	test marketing	0.75	4 October 1974
	endive (prepared, cut)	shelf-life extension	test marketing	1	14 January 1975
	onions	sprout inhibition	unconditional	0.05 max.	9 June 1975
	spices	decontamination	provisional	10	26 June 1975
	peeled potatoes	shelf-life extension	test marketing	0.5	12 May 1976
	chicken	shelf-life extension/decontamination	unconditional	3 max.	10 May 1976
	shrimps	shelf-life extension	test marketing	1	15 June 1976
	fillets of haddock, coal-fish, whiting	shelf-life extension	test marketing	1	6 September 1976
	fillets of cod and plaice	shelf-life extension	test marketing	1	7 September 1976
	fresh vegetables (prepared, cut, soup greens)	shelf-life extension	test marketing	1	6 September 1977

67

Food irradiation

Country	Product	Purpose of irradiation	Type of clearance	Dose permitted (kGy)	Date of approval
Netherlands (contd)	spices	decontamination	provisional	10	4 April 1978
	frozen frog legs	decontamination	provisional	5	25 September 1978
	rice and ground rice products	insect disinfestation	provisional	1	15 March 1979
	rye bread	shelf-life extension	provisional	5 max.	12 February 1980
	spices	decontamination	provisional	7 max.	15 April 1980
	frozen shrimp	decontamination	provisional	7 max.	9 May 1980
	malt	decontamination	provisional	10 max.	8 February 1983
	boiled and cooled shrimp	shelf-life extension	provisional	1 max.	8 February 1983
	frozen shrimp	decontamination	provisional	7 max.	8 February 1983
	frozen fish	decontamination	provisional	6 max.	24 August 1983
	egg powder	decontamination	provisional	6 max.	25 August 1983
	dry blood protein	decontamination	provisional	7 max.	25 August 1983
	dehydrated vegetables	decontamination	provisional	10 max.	27 October 1983
	refrigerated snacks of minced meat	shelf-life extension	test marketing	2	12 July 1984
New Zealand	herbs and spices (one batch)	decontamination	provisional	8	March 1985
Norway	spices	decontamination	unconditional	up to 10	
Philippines	potatoes	sprout inhibition	provisional	0.15 max.	13 September 1972
	onions	sprout inhibition	provisional	0.07	1981
	garlic	sprout inhibition	provisional	0.07	1981
	onions and garlic	sprout inhibition	test marketing		9 July 1984
Poland	potatoes	sprout inhibition	provisional	up to 0.15	1982
	onions	sprout inhibition	provisional		March 1983
Republic of Korea	potatoes	sprout inhibition	unconditional	0.15 max.	28 September 1987
	onions	sprout inhibition	unconditional	0.15 max.	28 September 1987
	garlic	sprout inhibition	unconditional	0.15 max.	28 September 1987
	chestnuts	sprout inhibition	unconditional	0.25 max.	28 September 1987
	fresh and dried mushrooms	growth inhibition/insect disinfestation	unconditional	1.00 max.	28 September 1987
South Africa	potatoes	sprout inhibition	unconditional	0.12–0.24	19 January 1977
	dried bananas	insect disinfestation	provisional	0.5 max.	28 July 1977
	avocados	insect disinfestation	provisional	0.1 max.	28 July 1977
	onions	sprout inhibition	unconditional	0.05–0.15	25 August 1978

Annex 1

Country	Product	Purpose of irradiation	Type of clearance	Dose permitted (kGy)	Date of approval
	garlic	sprout inhibition	unconditional	0.1–0.20	25 August 1978
	chicken	shelf-life extension/decontamination	unconditional	2–7	25 August 1978
	papaya	shelf-life extension	unconditional	0.5–1.5	25 August 1978
	mango	shelf-life extension	unconditional	0.5–1.5	25 August 1978
	strawberries	shelf-life extension	unconditional	1–4	25 August 1978
	bananas	shelf-life extension	unconditional		1982
	litchis	shelf-life extension	unconditional		1982
	pickled mango (achar)	shelf-life extension	unconditional		1982
	avocados	shelf-life extension	unconditional		1982
	frozen fruit juices	shelf-life extension	unconditional		
	green beans	shelf-life extension	unconditional		
	tomatoes	control of ripening	unconditional		
	brinjals		unconditional		
	soya pickle products		unconditional		
	ginger		unconditional		
	vegetable paste		unconditional		
	bananas (dried)	insect disinfestation	unconditional		
	almonds	insect disinfestation	unconditional		
	cheese powder	insect disinfestation	unconditional		
	yeast powder		unconditional		
	herbal tea		unconditional		
	various spices		unconditional		
	various dehydrated vegetables		unconditional		
Spain	potatoes	sprout inhibition	unconditional	0.05–0.15	4 November 1969
	onions	sprout inhibition	unconditional	0.08 max.	1971
Thailand	onions	sprout inhibition	unconditional	0.1 max.	20 March 1973
	potatoes, onions, garlic	sprout inhibition	unconditional	0.15	4 December 1986
	dates	disinfestation	unconditional	1	4 December 1986
	mangoes, papaya	disinfestation/delay of ripening	unconditional	1	4 December 1986
	wheat, rice, pulses	disinfestation	unconditional	1	4 December 1986
	cocoa beans	disinfestation	unconditional	1	4 December 1986
	fish and fishery products	reduce microbial load	unconditional	2.2	4 December 1986
	fish and fishery products	shelf-life extension	unconditional	3	4 December 1986
	strawberries	decontamination	unconditional	4	4 December 1986
	nam	decontamination	unconditional	5	4 December 1986
	moo yor	decontamination	unconditional	5	4 December 1986
	sausage	decontamination	unconditional	5	4 December 1986
	frozen shrimps		unconditional	5	4 December 1986
	cocoa beans	reduce microbial load	unconditional	5	4 December 1986

Food irradiation

Country	Product	Purpose of irradiation	Type of clearance	Dose permitted (kGy)	Date of approval
Thailand *(contd)*	chicken	decontamination/shelf-life extension	unconditional	7	4 December 1986
	spices & condiments, dehydrated	insect disinfestation	unconditional	1	4 December 1986
	onions and onion powder	decontamination	unconditional	10	4 December 1986
Union of Soviet Socialist Republics	potatoes	sprout inhibition	unconditional	0.1 max.	14 March 1958
	potaotes	sprout inhibition	unconditional	0.3 (1 MeV-electrons)	17 July 1973
	grain	insect disinfestation	unconditional	0.3	1959
	fresh fruits and vegetables	shelf-life extension	experimental batches	2–4	11 July 1964
	semi-prepared raw beef, pork & rabbit products (in plastic bags)	shelf-life extension	experimental batches	6–8	11 July 1964
	dried fruits	insect disinfestation	unconditional	1	15 February 1966
	dry food concentrates (buckwheat mush, gruel, rice, pudding)	insect disinfestation	unconditional	0.7	6 June 1966
	poultry, eviscerated (in plastic bags)	shelf-life extension	experimental batches	6	4 July 1966
	culinary prepared meat products (fried meat, entrecote) (in plastic bags)	shelf-life extension	test marketing	8	1 February 1967
	onions	sprout inhibition	test marketing	0.06	25 February 1967
	onions	sprout inhibition	unconditional	0.06	17 July 1973
United Kingdom	any food for consumption by patients who require a sterile diet as an essential factor in their treatment	sterilization	hospital patients		1 December 1969
United States of America	wheat and wheat flour	insect disinfestation	unconditional	0.2–0.5	21 August 1963
	white potatoes	shelf-life extension	unconditional	0.05–0.1	30 June 1964
	white potatoes	shelf-life extension	unconditional	0.05–0.15	1 November 1965
	spices and dry vegetable seasonings (38 commodities)	decontamination/insect disinfestation	unconditional	30 max.	5 July 1983
	dry or dehydrated enzyme preparations (including immobilized enzyme preparations)	control of insects and/or micro-organisms	unconditional	10 kGy max.	10 June 1985

Annex 1

Country	Product	Purpose of irradiation	Type of clearance	Dose permitted (kGy)	Date of approval
	pork carcasses or fresh, non-heat processed cuts of pork carcasses	control of *Trichinella spiralis*	unconditional	0.3 min. – 1.0 max.	22 July 1985
	fresh foods	delay or maturation	unconditional	1	18 April 1986
	food	disinfestation	unconditional	1	18 April 1986
	dry or dehydrated enzyme preparations	decontamination	unconditional	10	18 April 1986
	dry or dehydrated aromatic vegetable substances	decontamination	unconditional	30	18 April 1986
Uruguay	potatoes	sprout inhibition	unconditional		23 June 1970
Yugoslavia	cereals	insect disinfestation	unconditional	up to 10	17 December 1984
	legumes	insect disinfestation	unconditional	up to 10	17 December 1984
	onions	sprout inhibition	unconditional	up to 10	17 December 1984
	garlic	sprout inhibition	unconditional	up to 10	17 December 1984
	potatoes	sprout inhibition	unconditional	up to 10	17 December 1984
	dehydrated fruits & vegetables	sprout inhibition	unconditional	up to 10	17 December 1984
	dried mushrooms		unconditional	up to 10	17 December 1984
	egg powder	decontamination	unconditional	up to 10	17 December 1984
	herbal teas, tea extracts	decontamination	unconditional	up to 10	17 December 1984
	fresh poultry	shelf-life extension/decontamination	unconditional	up to 10	17 December 1984

Recommendations published by international organizations

Country	Product	Purpose of irradiation	Type of clearance	Dose permitted (kGy)	Date of approval
FAO/IAEA/WHO Expert Committee 1969	potatoes	sprout inhibition	provisional	0.15 max.	12 April 1969
	wheat and ground wheat products	insect disinfestation	provisional	0.75 max.	12 April 1969
FAO/IAEA/WHO Expert Committee 1976	potatoes	sprout inhibition	unconditional	0.03–0.15	7 September 1976
	onions	sprout inhibition	provisional	0.02–0.15	7 September 1976
	papaya	insect disinfestation	unconditional	0.5–1	7 September 1976
	strawberries	shelf-life extension	unconditional	1–3	7 September 1976
	wheat and ground wheat products	insect disinfestation	unconditional	0.15–1	7 September 1976
	rice	insect disinfestation	provisional	0.1–1	7 September 1976
	chicken	shelf-life extension/decontamination	unconditional	2–7	7 September 1976
	cod & redfish	shelf-life extension/decontamination	provisional	2–2.2	7 September 1976
FAO/IAEA/WHO Expert Committee 1980	any food product	sprout inhibition/shelf-life extension/decontamination insect disinfestation/control of ripening/growth inhibition	unconditional	up to 10	3 November 1980

Annex 2

CODEX GENERAL STANDARD FOR IRRADIATED FOODS[1]
(Worldwide Standard)

1. **Scope**

    This standard applies to foods processed by irradiation. It does not apply to foods exposed to doses imparted by measuring instruments used for inspection purposes.

2. **General requirements for the process**

    2.1 *Radiation sources*

    The following types of ionizing radiation may be used:

    (*a*) gamma rays from the radionuclides ^{60}Co or ^{137}Cs;

    (*b*) X-rays generated from machine sources operated at or below an energy level of 5 MeV;

    (*c*) electrons generated from machine sources operated at or below an energy level of 10 MeV.

    2.2 *Absorbed dose*

    The overall average dose absorbed by a food subjected to radiation processing should not exceed 10 kGy.[2,3]

    2.3 *Facilities and control of the process*

    2.3.1 Radiation treatment of foods shall be carried out in facilities licensed and registered for this purpose by the competent national authority.

---

[1] From the Codex Alimentarius, Vol. XV, 1984.

[2] For measurement and calculation of the overall average dose absorbed see Annex A of the Recommended International Code of Practice for the Operation of Irradiation Facilities used for Treatment of Foods (CAC/RCP 19-1979, Rev. 1). This Annex is reproduced in Appendix A to Annex 3 of this book, page 78

[3] The wholesomeness of foods, irradiated so as to have absorbed an overall average dose of up to 10 kGy, is not impaired. In this context the term "wholesomeness" refers to safety for consumption of irradiated foods from the toxicological point of view. The
irradiation of foods up to an overall average dose of 10 kGy introduces no special nutritional or microbiological problems (see WHO Technical Report Series No. 659, 1981 — *Wholesomeness of irradiated foods:* report of a Joint FAO/IAEA/WHO Expert Committee).

2.3.2 The facilities shall be designed to meet the requirements of safety, efficacy and good hygienic practices of food processing.

2.3.3 The facilities shall be staffed by adequate, trained and competent personnel.

2.3.4 Control of the process within the facility shall include the keeping of adequate records including quantitative dosimetry.

2.3.5 Premises and records shall be open to inspection by appropriate national authorities.

2.3.6 Control should be carried out in accordance with the Recommended International Code of Practice for the Operation of Radiation Facilities used for the Treatment of Foods (CAC/RCP 19-1979, Rev. 1).

3. Hygiene of irradiated foods

3.1 The food should comply with the provisions of the Recommended International Code of Practice — General Principles of Food Hygiene (Ref. No. CAC/RCP 1-1969, Rev. 1, 1979) and, where appropriate, with the Recommended International Code of Hygienic Practice of the Codex Alimentarius relative to a particular food.

3.2 Any relevant national public health requirement affecting microbiological safety and nutritional adequacy applicable in the country in which the food is sold should be observed.

4. Technological requirements

4.1 *Conditions for irradiation*

The irradiation of food is justified only when it fulfils a technological need or where it serves a food hygiene purpose[1] and should not be used as a substitute for good manufacturing practices.

4.2 *Food quality and packaging requirements*

The doses applied shall be commensurate with the technological and public health purposes to be achieved and shall be in accordance with good radiation processing practice. Foods to be

---

[1] The utility of the irradiation process has been demonstrated for a number of food items listed in Annex B to the Recommended International Code of Practice for the Operation of Irradiation Facilities used for the Treatment of Foods — CAC/RCP 19-1979 (Rev. 1). This Annex is reproduced in Appendix B to Annex 3 of this book (page 80)

irradiated and their packaging materials shall be of suitable quality, acceptable hygienic condition and appropriate for this purpose and shall be handled, before and after irradiation, according to good manufacturing practices taking into account the particular requirements of the technology of the process.

5. Re-irradiation

5.1 Except for foods with low moisture content (cereals, pulses, dehydrated foods and other such commodities) irradiated for the purpose of controlling insect reinfestation, foods irradiated in accordance with sections 2 and 4 of this standard shall not be re-irradiated.

5.2 For the purpose of this standard, food is not considered as having been re-irradiated when: (*a*) the food prepared from materials which have been irradiated at low dose levels, e.g., about 1 kGy, is irradiated for another technological purpose; (*b*) the food, containing less than 5% of irradiated ingredient, is irradiated, or when (*c*) the full dose of ionizing radiation required to achieve the desired effect is applied to the food in more than one instalment as part of processing for a specific technological purpose.

5.3 The cumulative overall average dose absorbed should not exceed 10 kGy as a result of re-irradiation.

6. Labelling

6.1 *Inventory control*

For irradiated foods, whether prepackaged or not, the relevant shipping documents shall give appropriate information to identify the registered facility which has irradiated the food, the date(s) of treatment and lot identification.

6.2 *Prepackaged foods intended for direct consumption*

The labelling of prepackaged irradiated foods shall be in accordance with the relevant provisions of the Codex General Standard for the Labelling of Prepackaged Foods.[1]

6.3 *Foods in bulk containers*

The declaration of the fact of irradiation shall be made clear on the relevant shipping documents.

---

[1] Under revision by the Codex Committee on Food Labelling.

Annex 3

RECOMMENDED INTERNATIONAL CODE OF PRACTICE FOR THE OPERATION OF IRRADIATION FACILITIES USED FOR THE TREATMENT OF FOOD[1]

1. **Introduction**

    This code refers to the operation of irradiation facilities based on the use of either a radionuclide source (^{60}Co or ^{137}Cs) or X-rays and electrons generated from machine sources. The irradiation facility may be of two designs, either "continuous" or "batch" type. Control of the food irradiation process in all types of facility involves the use of accepted methods of measuring the absorbed radiation dose and of the monitoring of the physical parameters of the process. The operation of these facilities for the irradiation of food must comply with the Codex recommendations on food hygiene.

2. **Irradiation plants**

   2.1 *Parameters*

    For all types of facility the doses absorbed by the product depend on the radiation parameter, the dwell time or the transportation speed of the product, and the bulk density of the material to be irradiated. Source–product geometry, especially distance of the product from the source and measures to increase the efficiency of radiation utilization, will influence the absorbed dose and the homogeneity of dose distribution.

   2.1.1 *Radionuclide sources*

    Radionuclides used for food irradiation emit photons of characteristic energies. The statement of the source material completely determines the penetration of the emitted radiation. The source activity is measured in becquerels (Bq) and should be stated by the supplying organization. The actual activity of the source (as well as any return or replenishment of radionuclide material) shall be recorded. The recorded activity should take into account the natural decay rate of the source and should be accompanied by a record of the date of measurement or

---

[1] From the *Codex Alimentarius*, Vol. XV, 1984.

recalculation. Radionuclide irradiators will usually have a well separated and shielded depository for the source elements and a treatment area which can be entered when the source is in the safe position. There should be a positive indication of the correct operational position and of the correct safe position of the source, which should be interlocked with the product movement system.

2.1.2 Machine sources

A beam of electrons generated by a suitable accelerator, or after being converted to X-rays, can be used. The penetration of the radiation is governed by the energy of the electrons. Average beam power shall be adequately recorded. There should be a positive indication of the correct setting of all machine parameters which should be interlocked with the product movement system. Usually a beam scanner or a scattering device (e.g., the converting target) is incorporated in a machine source to obtain an even distribution of the radiation over the surface of the product. The product movement, the width and speed of the scan and the beam pulse frequency (if applicable) should be adjusted to ensure a uniform surface dose.

2.2 Dosimetry and process control

Prior to the irradiation of any foodstuff certain dosimetry measurements[1] should be made, which demonstrate that the process will satisfy the regulatory requirements. Various techniques for dosimetry pertinent to radionuclide and machine sources are available for measuring absorbed dose in a quantitative manner.[2]

Dosimetry commissioning measurements should be made for each new food, irradiation process and whenever modifications are made to source strength or type and to the source–product geometry.

Routine dosimetry should be made during operation and records kept of such measurement. In addition, regular measurements of facility parameters governing the process, such as transportation speed, dwell time, source exposure time, machine beam parameters, can be made during the facility operation. The records of these measurements can be used as supporting evidence that the process satisfies the regulatory requirements.

3. Good radiation processing practice

Facility design should attempt to optimalize the dose uniformity ratio, to ensure appropriate dose rates and, where necessary, to

---

[1] See Appendix A to this Annex.

[2] Detailed in the *Manual of food irradiation dosimetry*. Vienna, IAEA, 1977 (Technical Report Series No. 178).

permit temperature control during irradiation (e.g., for the treatment of frozen food) and also control of the atmosphere. It is also often necessary to minimize mechanical damage to the product during transportation, irradiation and storage, and desirable to ensure the maximum efficiency in the use of the irradiator. Where the food to be irradiated is subject to special standards for hygiene or temperature control, the facility must permit compliance with these standards.

4. **Product and inventory control**

4.1 The incoming product should be physically separated from the outgoing irradiated products.

4.2 Where appropriate, a visual colour change radiation indicator should be affixed to each product pack for ready identification of irradiated and non-irradiated products.

4.3 Records should be kept in the facility record book which show the nature and kind of the product being treated, its identifying marks if packed or, if not, the shipping details, its bulk density, the type of source or electron machine, the dosimetry, the dosimeters used and details of their calibration, and the date of treatment.

4.4 All products shall be handled, before and after irradiation, according to accepted good manufacturing practices taking into account the particular requirements of the technology of the process[1]. Suitable facilities for refrigerated storage may be required.

---

[1] See Appendix B to this Annex.

Appendix A

Dosimetry

1. **The overall average absorbed dose**

   It can be assumed, for the purpose of the determination of the wholesomeness of food treated with an overall average dose of 10 kGy or less, that all radiation chemical effects in that particular dose range are proportional to dose.

   The overall average dose, $\overline{D}$, is defined by the following integral over the total volume of the goods:

   $$\overline{D} = \frac{1}{M} \int \rho(x, y, z) \cdot d(x, y, z) \cdot dV$$

   where:

   M = the total mass of the treated sample;
   ρ = the local density at the point (x, y, z);
   d = the local absorbed dose at the point (x, y, z);
   dV = $dx\, dy\, dz$ the infinitesimal volume element which in real cases is represented by the volume fractions.

   The overall average absorbed dose can be determined directly for homogeneous products or for bulk goods of homogeneous bulk density by distributing an adequate number of dose meters strategically and at random throughout the volume of the goods. From the dose distribution determined in this manner an average can be calculated which is the overall average absorbed dose.

   If the shape of the dose distribution curve through the product is well determined the positions of minimum and maximum dose are known. Measurements of the distribution of dose in these two positions in a series of samples of the product can be used to give an estimate of the overall average dose. In some cases the mean value of the average values of the minimum ($\overline{D}min$) and maximum ($\overline{D}max$) dose will be a good estimate of the overall average dose.

   Therefore in these cases:

   $$\text{overall average dose} \approx \frac{\overline{D}max + \overline{D}min}{2}$$

Annex 3

2. **Effective and limiting dose values**

   Some effective treatments, e.g., the elimination of harmful microorganisms, or a particular shelf-life extension, or a disinfestation, require a minimum absorbed dose. For other applications too high an absorbed dose may cause undesirable effects or an impairment of the quality of the product.

   The design of the facility and the operational parameters have to take into account minimum and maximum dose values required by the process. In some low dose applications it will be possible within the terms of section 3 on Good Radiation Processing Practice [see page 76] to allow a ratio of maximum to minimum dose of greater than 3.

   With regards to the maximum dose value under acceptable wholesomeness considerations, and because of the statistical distribution of the dose, a mass fraction of product of at least 97.5% should receive an absorbed dose of less than 15 kGy when the overall average dose is 10 kGy.

3. **Routine dosimetry**

   Measurements of the dose in a reference position can be made occasionally throughout the process. The association between the dose in the reference position and the overall average dose must be known. These measurements should be used to ensure the correct operation of the process. A recognized and calibrated system of dosimetry should be used.

   A complete record of all dosimetry measurements including calibration must be kept.

4. **Process control**

   In the case of a continuous radionuclide facility it will be possible to make automatically a record of transportation speed or dwell time together with indications of source and product positioning. These measurements can be used to provide a continuous control of the process in support of routine dosimetry measurements.

   In a batch-operated radionuclide facility, automatic recording of source exposure time can be made and a record of product movement and placement can be kept to provide a control of the process in support of routine dosimetry measurements.

   In a machine facility, a continuous record of beam parameters, e.g., voltage, current, scan speed, scan width, pulse repetition and a record of transportation speed through the beam, can be used to provide a continuous control of the process in support of routine dosimetry measurements.

Appendix B

Examples of technological conditions for the irradiation of some individual food items specifically examined by the Joint FAO/IAEA/WHO Expert Committee

This information is taken from the reports of the Joint FAO/IAEA/WHO Expert Committee on Food Irradiation (WHO Technical Report Series, No. 604, 1977 and No. 659, 1981) and illustrates the utility of the irradiation process. It also describes the technical conditions for achieving the purpose of the irradiation process safely and economically.

1. Chicken (*Gallus domesticus*)

1.1 *Purposes of the process*

The purposes of irradiating chicken are:

(*a*) to prolong storage life;

(*b*) to reduce the number of certain pathogenic microorganisms, such as *Salmonella* from eviscerated chicken.

1.2 *Specific requirements*

1.2.1 *Average dose:* for (*a*) and (*b*), up to 7 kGy.

2. Cocoa beans (*Theobroma cacao*)

2.1 *Purposes of the process*

The purposes of irradiating cocoa beans are:

(*a*) to control insect infestation in storage

(*b*) to reduce microbial load of fermented beans with or without heat treatment.

2.2 *Specific requirements*

2.2.1 *Average dose:* for (*a*) up to 1 kGy; for (*b*) up to 5 kGy.

Annex 3

2.2.2 *Prevention of reinfestation*

Cocoa beans, whether prepackaged or handled in bulk, should be stored as far as possible under such conditions as will prevent reinfestation and microbial recontamination and spoilage.

3. Dates (*Phoenix dactylifera*)

3.1 *Purpose of the process*

The purpose of irradiating prepackaged dried dates is to control insect infestation during storage.

3.2 *Specific requirements*

3.2.1 *Average dose:* up to 1 kGy.

3.2.2 *Prevention of reinfestation*

Prepackaged dried dates should be stored under such conditions as will prevent reinfestation.

4. Mangoes (*Mangifera indica*)

4.1 *Purposes of the process*

The purposes of irradiating mangoes are:
- (*a*) to control insect infestation;
- (*b*) to improve keeping quality by delaying ripening;
- (*c*) to reduce microbial load by combining irradiation and heat treatment.

4.2 *Specific requirements*

4.2.1 *Average dose:* up to 1 kGy.

5. Onions (*Allium cepa*)

5.1 *Purpose of the process*

The purpose of irradiating onions is to inhibit sprouting during storage.

5.2 *Specific requirement*

5.2.1 *Average dose:* up to 0.15 kGy.

6. Papaya (Carica papaya L.)

6.1 Purpose of the process

The purpose of irradiating papaya is to control insect infestation and to improve its keeping quality by delaying ripening.

6.2 Specific requirements

6.2.1 *Average dose:* up to 1 kGy.

6.2.2 *Source of radiation*

The source of radiation should be such as will provide adequate penetration.

7. Potatoes (Solanum tuberosum L.)

7.1 Purpose of the process

The purpose of irradiating potatoes is to inhibit sprouting during storage.

7.2 Specific requirement

7.2.1 *Average dose:* up to 0.15 kGy.

8. Pulses

8.1 Purpose of the process

The purpose of irradiating pulses is to control insect infestation in storage.

8.2 Specific requirement

8.2.1 *Average dose:* up to 1 kGy.

9. Rice (Oriza species)

9.1 Purpose of the process

The purpose of irradiating rice is to control insect infestation in storage.

9.2 Specific requirements

9.2.1 *Average dose:* up to 1 kGy.

Annex 3

9.2.2 *Prevention of reinfestation*

Rice, whether prepackaged or handled in bulk, should be stored, as far as possible, under such conditions as will prevent reinfestation.

10. Spices and condiments, dehydrated onions, onion powder

10.1 *Purposes of the process*

The purposes of irradiating spices, condiments, dehydrated onions and onion powder are:

(*a*) to control insect infestation;

(*b*) to reduce microbial load;

(*c*) to reduce the number of pathogenic microorganisms.

10.2 *Specific requirement*

10.2.1 *Average dose:* for (*a*) up to 1 kGy;
for (*b*) and (*c*) up to 10 kGy.

11. Strawberry (*Fragaria* species)

11.1 *Purpose of the process*

The purpose of irradiating fresh strawberries is to prolong the storage life by partial elimination of spoilage organisms.

11.2 *Specific requirement*

11.2.1 *Average dose:* up to 3 kGy.

12. Teleost fish and fish products

12.1 *Purposes of the process*

The purposes of irradiating teleost fish and fish products are:

(*a*) to control insect infestation of dried fish during storage and marketing;

(*b*) to reduce microbial load of the packaged or unpackaged fish and fish products;

(*c*) to reduce the number of certain pathogenic microorganisms in packaged or unpackaged fish and fish products.

12.2   *Specific requirements*

12.2.1 *Average dose:* for (*a*) up to 1 kGy;
        for (*b*) and (*c*) up to 2.2 kGy.

12.2.2 *Temperature requirement*

During irradiation and storage the fish and fish products referred to in (*b*) and (*c*) should be kept at the temperature of melting ice.

13. Wheat and ground wheat products (*Triticum* species)

13.1   *Purpose of the process*

The purpose of irradiating wheat and ground wheat products is to control insect infestation in the stored product.

13.2   *Specific requirements*

13.2.1 *Average dose:* up to 1 kGy.

13.2.2 *Prevention of reinfestation*

These products, whether prepackaged or handled in bulk, should be stored as far as possible under such conditions as will prevent reinfestation.